Make Your Own

PURE MINERAL MAKEUP

79 easy hypoallergenic recipes
for radiant beauty

HEATHER ANDERSON

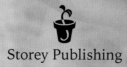

Storey Publishing

The mission of Storey Publishing is to serve our customers by publishing practical information that encourages personal independence in harmony with the environment.

Edited by Gwen Steege and Michal Lumsden
Art direction and book design by Alethea Morrison
Text production by Jennifer Jepson Smith
Indexed by Christine R. Lindemer, Boston Road Communications

Cover and interior photography by **Mars Vilaubi**, front cover, 3, 14, 30, 31, 38, 47, 50, 53, 56, 59, 60, 65–74, 83, 85, 86, 88–90, 92–94, 96, 97, 99, 100, 102–104, 106–108, 110–112, 114–118, 120–124, 126–130, 132, 142–146, 148–152, 154–164, 166–170, 172–178, 184–186, 188, 190, 192–194, 198 (middle right and bottom) and © **Melinda DiMauro**, back cover, 1, 4, 6, 11, 27, 33, 35, 44, 49, 79, 87, 91, 95, 98, 101, 105, 109, 113, 119, 125, 131, 133, 147, 153, 165, 171, 179, 182, 187, 191, 195, 198 (left and top right), 202–208, 214, 218, 226, 228
Additional photography by © 1995 Harry Langdon/Getty Images, 212 (Diana); © 2011 Gamma-Rapho/Getty Images, 213 (Brigitte); © 2012 Getty Images, 212 (Bette); © Alfred Eisenstaedt/Getty Images, 213 (Marilyn); © Arif Iqball Photography-Japan/Alamy Stock Photos, 19 (right); © Bettmann Archive/Getty images, 213 (Clara); © Donaldson Collection/Getty Images, 213 (Greta); © Graphic Arts/Getty Images, 20 (left); © Heather Anderson, 250; © InFocus/Alamy Stock Photos, 19 (left); © John Kobal Foundation/Getty Images, 212 (Audrey); John Polak, 8, 22, 36, 54, 62, 76, 196, 220; © Keystone Features/Getty Images, 212 (Sophia); © Lipnitzki/Roger Viollet/Getty Images, 17; © Michael Putland/Getty Images, 21 (right); © popper foto/Getty Images, 21 (left); © Silver Screen Collection/Getty Images, 18, 20 (right)
Illustrations by © Samantha Hahn, except 226 by © Heather Anderson

© 2017 by Heather Anderson

Be sure to read all the instructions thoroughly before undertaking any of the projects in this book and follow all the safety guidelines provided. Please consult with your doctor before use. The makeup made using the recipes in this book is for personal use only; commercial use of the recipes is forbidden without permission of the author.

The information in this book is true and complete to the best of our knowledge. All recommendations are made without guarantee on the part of the author or Storey Publishing. The author and publisher disclaim any liability in connection with the use of this information.

Storey books are available for special premium and promotional uses and for customized editions. For further information, please call 800-793-9396.

Storey Publishing
210 MASS MoCA Way
North Adams, MA 01247
storey.com

Printed in China by Toppan Leefung Printing Ltd.
10 9 8 7 6 5 4 3 2 1

LIBRARY OF CONGRESS CATALOGING-IN-PUBLICATION DATA ON FILE

This book is dedicated
to my two sweet girls,
who are the definition of beauty
and goodness, and
to all the unique
unexpected beauties
of the world.
Thank you for your
inspiration.

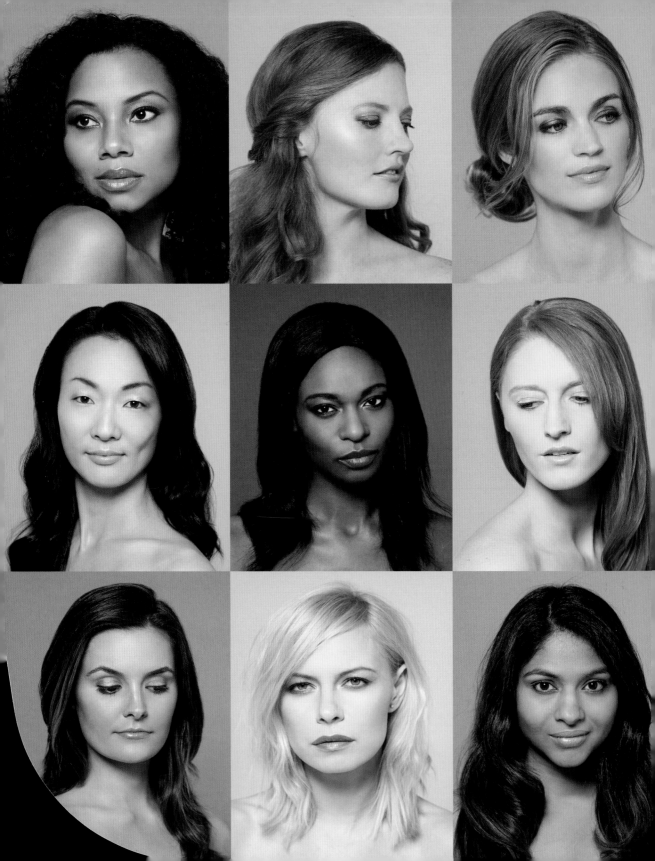

CONTENTS

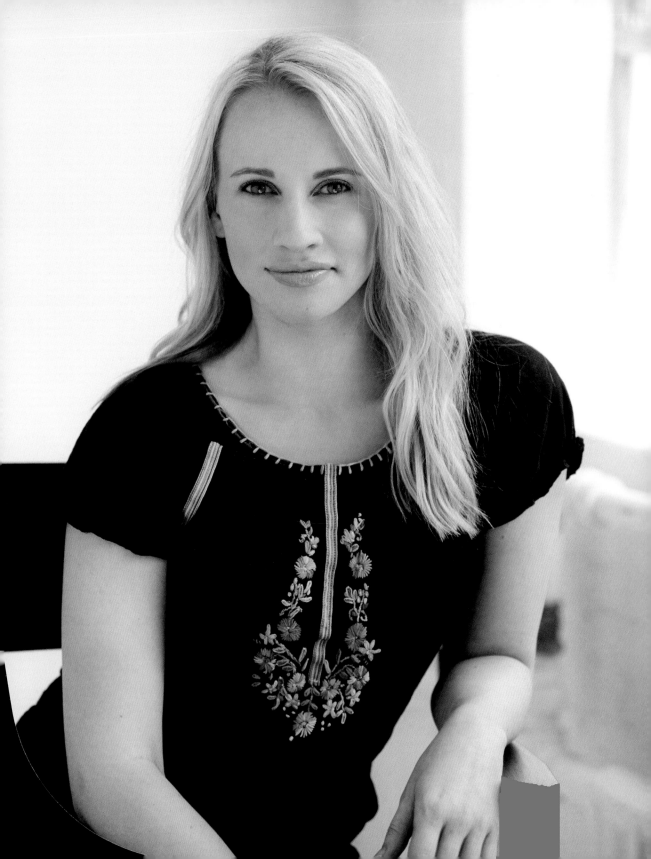

INTRODUCTION

For many years, I struggled with acne. I tried every home remedy, diet, over-the-counter spot treatment, and topical gel I could find, and even a few prescriptions. Nothing seemed to help. After seeing several dermatologists, I was diagnosed with perioral dermatitis and told that I would have to stop wearing any makeup containing chemicals or bismuth oxychloride, a common cosmetic ingredient.

My only makeup option was mineral makeup. I soon learned that mineral makeup can be rather expensive to buy, and many brands even contain bismuth oxychloride, so I searched for ways to make my own. I stumbled across a few blogs that listed recipes for organic homemade "mineral makeup." There wasn't much to the recipes, just combining a few spices with cornstarch. I mixed up my first batch and was excited to see that it looked just like store-bought mineral makeup. Then I smelled it, and tried it, and was immediately discouraged: the makeup was simple in theory but lacking in performance. These powders offered no coverage, and instead of blending into the skin to look natural, they created a powdery mask.

Eventually I found a company that sold not only mineral makeup products but also kits to make your own. I got an eye shadow kit and used up all the ingredients in the same week. I started creating my own recipes, experimenting with colors, and pressing my own eye shadows. When I shared pictures of my creations online, friends asked if they could buy them. I sold to friends and family for a year or so, then decided to expand and sell online. Investors and a crowd-funding website helped me start my company, Kaleidoscope Cosmetics. From there I started selling online and in a local boutique.

Because of the lack of information available on creating mineral makeup, I eventually decided to write a book, sharing my recipes and knowledge with those interested in crafting their own. I hope you find the result educational and fun!

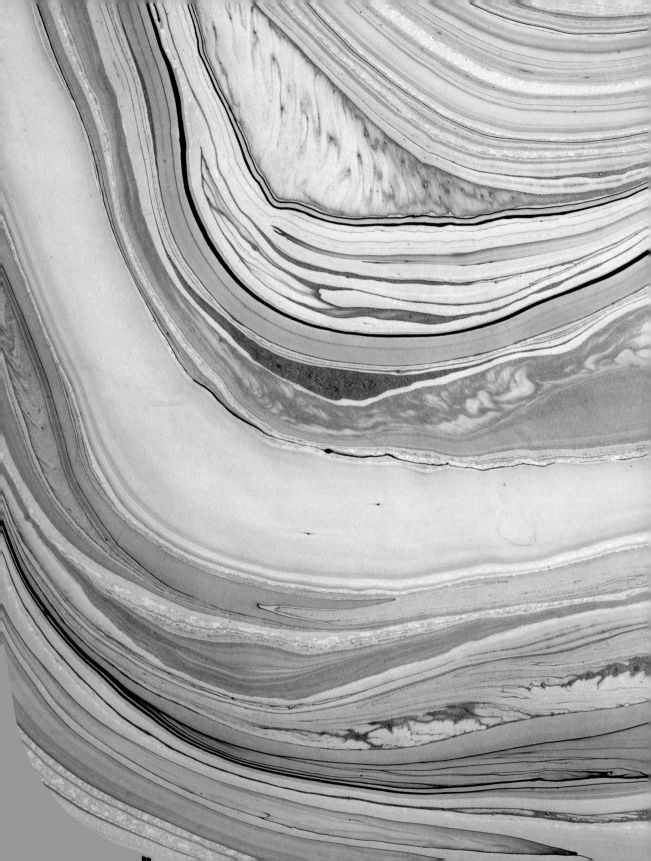

CHAPTER 1

WHY MINERAL MAKEUP?

Some of us get dipped in flat, some in satin, some in gloss. . . . But every once in a while, you find someone who's iridescent, and when you do, nothing will ever compare.

WENDELIN VAN DRAANEN

Makeup is not a modern novelty. People have been decorating their bodies with clays, paints, and dyes for centuries. Mineral makeup as we know it today, however, is a more recent innovation. In the early 1970s, after shopping at a small body-care shop in Rice Village, a trendy outdoor mall in Houston, kindergarten teacher Diane Richardson Ranger was inspired to start making her own body products. She had no experience formulating cosmetics, but her enthusiasm and commitment led her to open her own body-care boutique in Northern California. Ranger saw a need for more natural body-care products and wanted to create makeup products free of what she called the "seven deadly skins": perfume, talc, alcohol, mineral oil, preservatives, emulsifiers, and dyes. In 1976 she founded Bare Escentuals, the first modern mineral makeup brand. In the four decades since, she has started several more mineral makeup companies, and still others have popped up around the globe.

At the same time that Ranger was starting Bare Escentuals, the fields of dermatology and plastic surgery were evolving. Invasive treatments like chemical peels, microdermabrasion, laser skin resurfacing, and waxing became routine. These procedures can diminish signs of aging and treat some skin conditions, but they also can leave patients' skin raw for a couple days to a few weeks. Any makeup worn while the skin heals must be very gentle. Free of chemicals and irritants, mineral makeup can camouflage bruising from surgical procedures and redness or irritation from peels, burns, and waxing. Because mineral makeup was the only safe option for women who wanted to wear cosmetics while healing, dermatologists and plastic surgeons played an important role in its rising popularity.

Interest in mineral makeup grew even more when the new CEO of Bare Escentuals began selling her products on a popular home shopping television network in the late 1990s. Soon she was selling $1.4 million worth of products an hour. Drugstores and department stores quickly joined the movement, creating their own versions of mineral makeup.

Not all mineral makeup is created equal, however. Many large-scale cosmetic brands sell "mineral makeup" lines that include irritants, synthetic and petroleum-based ingredients, and inexpensive fillers that create bulk but can also irritate the skin. Many of these products also contain waxes, oils, dyes, and preservatives.

The more ingredients a product contains, the higher the risk of it causing a skin irritation or allergy.

What distinguishes mineral makeup from most mainstream makeup is what is *left out* rather than what is added. True mineral makeup has fewer ingredients than traditional commercially produced makeup — and all of those ingredients are derived from naturally occurring materials. Today many of these ingredients are formulated in laboratories to ensure consistent colors and textures and to keep them free of potentially harmful impurities. They are chemically identical to what's found

Susannah is wearing

EYES: Cream Soda shadow; Chimney eyeliner; Blondie eyebrow powder

LIPS: Orange Sherbet

FACE: Vanilla foundation; Sun-Kissed bronzer; Sugar Peach blush; Wonderland highlighter

in nature, though, and makers of pure mineral cosmetics are careful not to add perfumes, dyes, or fillers that can irritate the skin and clog pores. Mineral makeup's oil-free loose powders sit on top of the skin instead of soaking in, as creams and liquids do. This helps keep pores unclogged and reduces the chance of irritation, which most often occurs when an ingredient is absorbed into the skin.

BENEFITS OF MINERAL MAKEUP

SAFE ingredients can be used on sensitive skin, acne-prone skin, injured skin, perioral dermatitis, and rosacea.

INERT ingredients are bacteria-free and won't expire.

EFFECTIVE ingredients help heal, soothe, and protect the skin.

NATURAL ingredients are free of potentially irritating chemicals, synthetics, fragrances, preservatives, parabens, gluten, oils, and waxes.

GENTLE ingredients promote healthy skin and won't clog pores.

VERSATILE pigments can be used wet or dry as a temporary hair colorant, lip color, blush, highlighter, eye shadow, eyeliner, and body shimmer.

COVERAGE is buildable from sheer to opaque.

FEWER ingredients mean less chance of irritation.

LONG-LASTING mixtures bind to the oils of your skin and are water resistant.

PROTECTS by creating a barrier between the skin, elements, and free radicals and can offer some sun protection.

BOTANICALS

Ingredients derived from plants are optional additions to mineral makeup formulations. I incorporate botanicals in some of my recipes because these plant-based ingredients offer some real benefits to the crafting process and to the final product. Botanicals can be used along with mineral ingredients or as a substitute for certain ingredients. Often these plant-based powders are less expensive than mineral powders, so incorporating them cuts down on the total cost of creating some mineral makeup products. In addition, some crafters like to test color-blend recipes with botanical powders like cornstarch as a cheaper way to experiment with new recipes. Certain botanical powders, such as rice powder and cornstarch, can be healing and soothing to the skin. The downside to using botanicals is that, unlike inert minerals, these plant-based ingredients can harbor and spread bacteria, and they can spoil or become rancid.

WHY MAKE YOUR OWN?

You now know what makes mineral makeup different from most store-bought cosmetics, but you may still wonder why you should make your own. There are many reasons.

IT'S CUSTOMIZABLE. When you mix your own ingredients, you can match your skin color perfectly. This is especially useful for people with very pale or dark skin shades. You can also tailor your handmade mixtures to best suit your skin type — whether it's normal, oily, dry, combination, or sensitive. Finally, choosing your own ingredients means you can create the precise finish and cover that will help you look your best. Do you want a foundation that shimmers slightly to give your skin a subtle glow? Or one that has a matte finish and can help heal and camouflage your acne at the same time? No problem.

YOU ARE IN CONTROL. Because you are the one preparing the recipes, you decide which ingredients to use. This gives you more control over the cost, color, and finish of each product. For example, the recipes in this book use only pure mineral and botanical powders. Although the U.S. Food and Drug

Administration allows many petroleum-based colorants in cosmetics, I prefer to avoid these ingredients. You can use the ingredients glossary (page 236) and some independent experimenting to tweak my recipes or make your own using the exact ingredients you want. In addition, when you choose to create mineral makeup, you can decide if you want to trade in all your old cosmetics or just pick certain products to craft, while continuing to buy others from the store. For instance, I produce almost all of my own cosmetics but haven't been able to formulate the perfect mascara recipe just yet, so for now I make everything I wear except mascara. Creating your own makeup doesn't have to be an all-or-nothing undertaking. Transitioning to higher-quality mineral cosmetics can help you live a healthier life, but you have to do what works best for you!

THE REWARDS GO DEEPER THAN YOUR SKIN. Your appearance is a part of how you express yourself. And what better way to do so than to handcraft your own look? It's a great way to show off your creativity, and the possibilities are endless. You don't have to limit yourself to what's trendy or to what you can buy in a store. Instead, you can mix and match trends and colors as you like, and you can experiment for lower-cost alternatives to your favorite product. Choosing your own ingredients also lets you craft products that mirror your belief system. You can create vegan makeup, steer clear of oils, and use recyclable containers. And the ultimate reward? When you make something you're proud of, you can give it away as a gift. Nothing is more gratifying than sharing something you've made with someone you love.

THE PLANET — AND YOUR CHILDREN — WILL REAP THE BENEFITS. Synthetic chemicals can harm both your face and the planet, but hand-mixing your own mineral makeup ensures that you can use only safe, natural ingredients. When you create your own cosmetics, you also embrace self-sufficiency. This small act can send a big message to the powerful beauty industry. By breaking with this part of consumer culture, you exercise your power to step away from dominant messages about what is considered "beautiful" and instead wear only the makeup you want, and how you want.

IT'S EASIER — AND CHEAPER — THAN YOU THINK. To get started, you need only a few ingredients and a handful of common kitchen tools. You do not need special training or a degree to create your own makeup; anyone can do it. Most recipes require just a couple steps, and the techniques are not difficult to learn. If you get hooked, you can buy some ingredients in bulk to significantly reduce your costs. Many of the final products share the same ingredients, so you'll have to purchase only a few items. The same ingredients you use to put together foundation, for example, will also make eyeliner, concealer, blush, bronzer, and highlighter. Even if you decide not to purchase in bulk, many of the ingredients are widely available online, so you can shop around for prices to meet your budget. One of the reasons I love preparing my own mineral makeup is because I save so much money. Instead of paying upwards of $20 for store-bought foundation, I can custom-blend my own for only a couple dollars! Instead of paying for the brand name, marketing, advertising, and production costs of a purchased product, you control the costs and choose what you want to spend money on.

MAKING AND SELLING MAKEUP ARE MARKETABLE SKILLS. If you are a makeup artist or an aesthetician, learning how to customize all-natural makeup could be a skill that sets you apart from your competition. Once you feel confident preparing makeup, you could turn your passion into a profitable business plan.

YOU'RE BEAUTIFUL

With popular culture and the media constantly bombarding us with their standards of beauty, it is important for each of us to remember to appreciate and care for ourselves. Natural beauty is about seeing ourselves as we truly are, not trying to change into someone else. We all have parts of ourselves we don't like. But instead of focusing on the negative, try to find what sets you apart from others and celebrate your differences. One of my favorite quotes is from the French fashion designer Coco Chanel, who said, "In order to be irreplaceable, you must always be different."

As I have developed my cosmetic company I have learned the importance of self-care, which is different from being selfish. Self-care is being compassionate and nurturing to yourself. The world sends mixed messages to women, expecting us to project a certain kind of beauty, yet shaming us for pursuing that standard — whether through plastic surgery, makeup, or dieting — by calling us vain, shallow, or insecure. To be sure, wearing makeup is not necessary, as everyone is beautiful just as we are, but wearing makeup can be a form of self-care. Makeup is a powerful tool that can accentuate our favorite features, enhance our natural beauty, and help us feel confident — and there is nothing wrong with that.

PRO TIP
MAKING MAKEUP, BUILDING SKILLS

If you are currently a makeup artist, or are training to become one, producing your own cosmetics will set you apart from your competition. You will be able to customize makeup to meet each of your clients' unique needs. When you go to a session, you can bring everything you'll need to mix up new eye shadows, lip colors, and other products on-site. If you don't have a color your client wants, you can whip it up in just a few minutes, providing your client with customizable support and the most gorgeous results.

Always include on your résumé and profiles your knowledge of creating mineral makeup, as well as any specific training or certifications you have completed. The skill alone may qualify you for a job.

Your style of grooming, whether that includes wearing makeup or not, is a personal choice. It's something you should do for yourself, not for others. Every morning as you get ready for the day, treat those minutes as a time to show yourself that you are important. Give it a try: you deserve to feel beautiful!

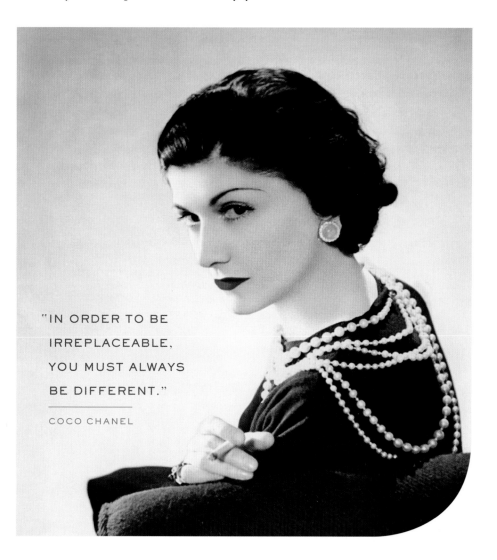

"IN ORDER TO BE
IRREPLACEABLE,
YOU MUST ALWAYS
BE DIFFERENT."

COCO CHANEL

GLAMOUR SNAPSHOTS IN TIME

Women and men have chosen to adorn and decorate themselves for millennia. While makeup production and styles have certainly evolved through the years, the desire to add to one's natural appearance has remained constant.

The earliest record of makeup starts in ancient Egypt, where Cleopatra lined her eyes with kohl, a mixture of many ingredients including ash, copper, and ocher. Common Egyptians also lined their eyes with this black powder to protect their eyes in the fields from the bright desert sun.

Women in ancient Greece wore a white face powder made of lead and used crushed mulberries as blush and lip stain. Light skin was also prized in the Roman Empire, and women used whitening powders made from lead and chalk. Rose

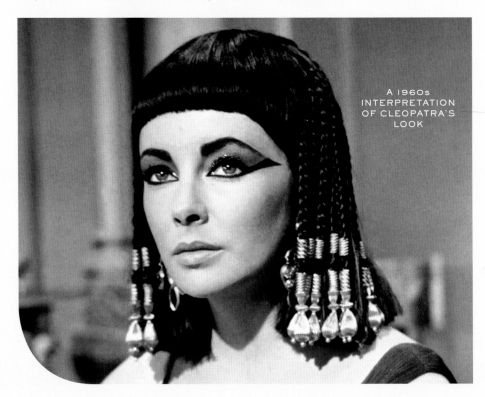

A 1960s
INTERPRETATION
OF CLEOPATRA'S
LOOK

petals, ocher, and wine were all used to make rouge, and eyelashes were darkened and thickened with a range of substances, including burnt cork and kohl.

Farther east, ancient Indians and Persians used henna to decorate their bodies, a tradition that continues to this day. It was common in ancient China to stain the fingernails with beeswax, egg, gelatin, and gum arabic, and beginning around AD 800, Japanese geishas painted their faces with powders made originally from white lead paint and later from rice powder. Geishas also outlined their eyes with charcoal and wore red lipstick made from safflower petals. In Australia, ceremonial face and body painting among aborigines is a centuries-old tradition used to help identify an individual's tribe, social status, family, and more. Historically the paint was pigmented with clay, feathers, ocher, and plant materials.

During the Middle Ages in Europe, pale skin was a sign of wealth, as tanned skin was often the result of working in the fields. Some women bled themselves to try to attain a pale complexion, while others created face masks with egg whites. Face paints and powders made of arsenic and lead were commonly

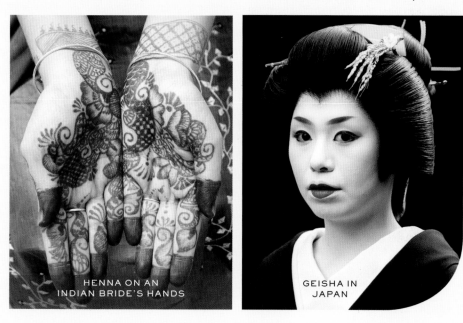

HENNA ON AN
INDIAN BRIDE'S HANDS

GEISHA IN
JAPAN

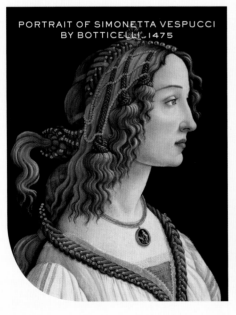

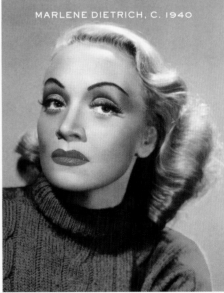

used throughout the Renaissance. When Queen Victoria declared makeup to be vulgar and improper, many English women stopped wearing it, though cosmetics remained common among actors and prostitutes.

Native American tribes traditionally painted their faces and bodies for battle as well as for spiritual ceremonies and dances. While each tribe used its own unique color combinations and patterns, every design meant something specific and conveyed information about the wearer's accomplishments, skills, social status, and the like. The paints were made from natural materials available in the area, including berries, clay, and minerals.

By the early 1900s in the United States, a pale, youthful complexion was the standard of beauty and many women wore some kind of makeup to achieve that look. Many cosmetics manufacturers had already stopped using the deadly ingredients that historically had been used in cosmetics — such as lead, arsenic, and mercury — and in 1902, Congress passed the Biologics Control Act, the first governmental regulation of cosmetics and related products.

PORTRAIT OF SIMONETTA VESPUCCI BY BOTTICELLI, 1475

MARLENE DIETRICH, C. 1940

Seven years later, an immigrant named Max Factor — who had served as the private beautician for Russia's royal family — moved to Los Angeles and started the first professional makeup company specifically for movie actors. His products made stars of the silver screen look realistic and natural, while still appearing glamorous. Bette Davis, Marlene Dietrich, and Jean Harlow were among Factor's most famous clients. He coined the term *make-up* and in 1920 unveiled the first standardized cosmetics line sold to the general public.

After World War II, numerous cosmetic brands were established in the United States as makeup became more mainstream. In part due to the growing feminist movement, many women decided to stop wearing makeup in the 1960s and 1970s. Others duplicated Twiggy's doe-eyed eyeliner and fake-lashes look. By the 1980s, extreme bright colors and an overly made-up look were fashionable. Today, as the world is ever more connected through technology, the idea of a single dominant makeup style has given way to multiple popular looks, many of which draw from diverse cultures.

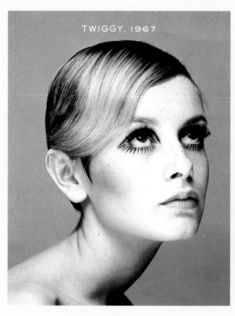

TWIGGY, 1967

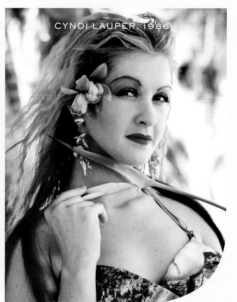

CYNDI LAUPER, 1986

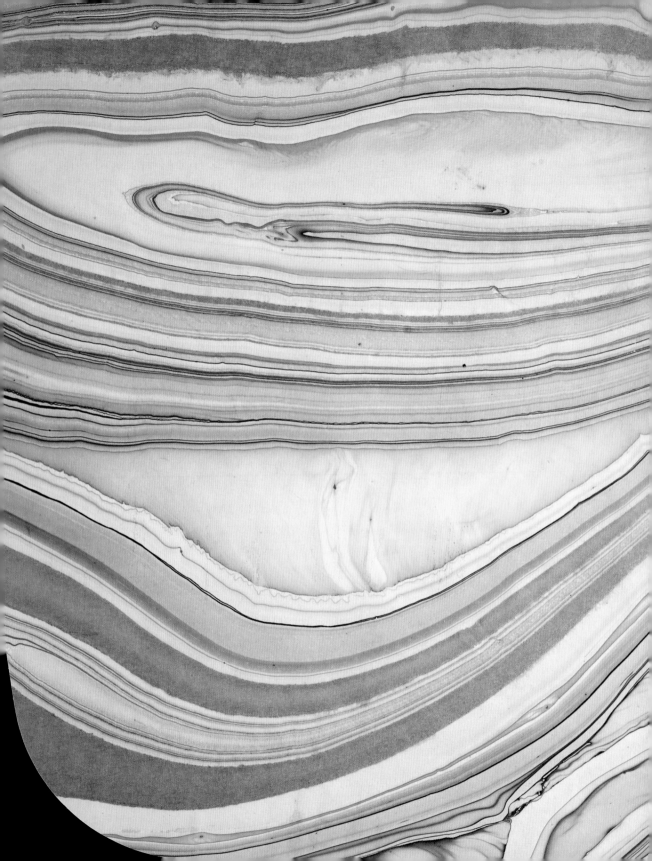

CHAPTER 2

ALL ABOUT COLOR

Sunset is still my favorite color, and rainbow is second.

MATTIE STEPANEK

Creating custom colors is one of the most exciting parts of making your own makeup, but it can also be one of the most intimidating. Understanding how to choose the right color for your skin color, shade, and undertone is key. I begin with basic color theory and later discuss mixing and selecting the perfect color for application.

These lessons can guide your decisions about which eye shadow, eyeliner, blush, lip gloss, bronzer, and highlighter recipes will not only look good with your eyes and hair but also work well together. A more subtle process — but equally, if not more, important — is using color theory to create foundation that matches your skin perfectly. This will ensure that you have a flawless palette on which to apply the rest of your makeup.

COLOR BASICS

Everyone sees and understands color a little differently, which makes verbal descriptions related to color confusing. I'll use some diagrams, therefore, to clarify these important points.

Sir Isaac Newton organized colors in the shape of a wheel, a tool that can help us see how colors are related to one another. In makeup, as well as in art or any other subject related to color, it is important to understand the basic rules and guidelines that aid in color mixing and picking out colors for a project. You will find yourself applying basic color theory concepts throughout your makeup journey.

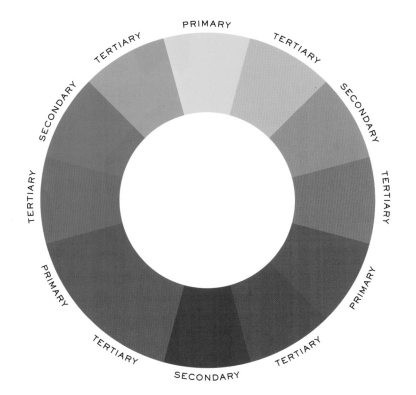

PRIMARY COLORS are red, yellow, and blue. With these three colors, you can create any other color.

SECONDARY COLORS are orange, green, and violet. They are made by mixing together two primary colors in equal proportions.

TERTIARY COLORS are produced by mixing a primary color with an adjacent secondary color. They have many names and variations; in the simplest terms, they include red orange, orange yellow, yellow green, green blue, blue violet, and violet red.

ANALOGOUS COLORS are any three colors that are next to each other on the color wheel. When choosing colors for a makeup look or an eye shadow palette, stick to colors that are close to one another on the color wheel. These colors are harmonious and look good together.

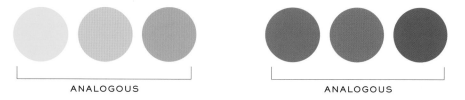

ANALOGOUS   ANALOGOUS

COMPLEMENTARY COLORS are directly across from each other on the color wheel. When choosing eye makeup, it is good to know what color complements your natural eye color. To enhance your eye color, or make your eyes "pop," choose colors that are located opposite your eye color on the color wheel.

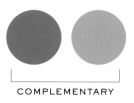

COMPLEMENTARY

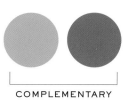

COMPLEMENTARY

MONOCHROMATIC refers to using only one hue, which can be made to look darker or lighter by shade, tint, and tone. If you want to ensure that all of your makeup matches and looks cohesive, you can stick to hues that are all in the same color family. For example, you could use tan and brown eye shadows, a nude lip color, and a medium bronze blush.

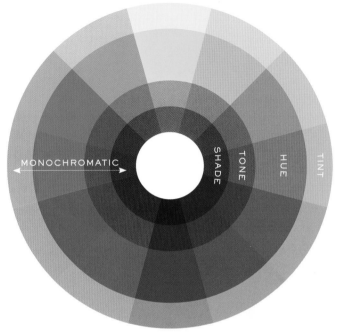

MORE COLOR DEFINITIONS

HUE. The color itself, such as red, orange, yellow, green, blue, or violet.

SATURATION. The intensity of a color, which is determined by how much hue is included.

TINT. Hue, with white added.

SHADE. Hue, with black added.

TONE. Hue, with gray added.

Nani is wearing

EYES: Chimney shadow; Chimney liner

LIPS: Basic Lip Gloss mixed with Vamp

FACE: Nutmeg–Cream Puff foundation mixture (50:50); Suede bronzer; Vamp blush; Buttercream highlighter

Applying Your Knowledge

Once you are familiar with color theory, you can play around with your recipes, palettes, and application. You will be surprised at how often you will use color theory when working with cosmetics. Use the color wheel to guide you when making and applying cosmetics.

Referring to the color wheel helps you know how to create specific colors and how to alter a color when it is not right. It is much easier to match hues, shades, and tints once you can spot the basic colors and any underlying hints of other incorporated colors. You will then be better equipped to masterfully mix colors, adding black to make a darker shade, adding white to make a tint lighter, and adding a complementary color to make the hue less saturated. Having a basic understanding of color theory can allow you to create millions of color blends.

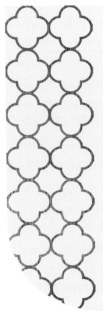

BEAUTY SPOT
CHOOSING COLORS

Whether you are making or applying cosmetics, choose colors that enhance beauty. Pay attention to your skin shade and undertones (pages 33–35), preferences, and hair and eye colors. If you have warm skin undertones, stick to earth tones like golds, bronze, reds, yellows, and oranges. If you have cool skin undertones, use silvers and grays, or bright and crisp jewel tones like green, blue, and violet. Draw attention to your natural eye color by choosing complementary tones. For example, if you have blue eyes, try an eye shadow color that is orange based, like copper; this will make your eyes stand out.

COSMETIC COLOR ADDITIVES

There are three primary ways that I add color to mineral makeup. Each lends different qualities to the final product, so it is important to understand these ingredients before you start mixing your own recipes.

PIGMENTS such as iron oxides are matte powders that give your mineral makeup dimension and color. While today many pigments are synthetically produced, they are based on the natural coloring matter of minerals, plants, or, occasionally, animals. Naturally derived versions of some pigments are available.

MICA is a lustrous mineral that is ground into a white powder, which can then be coated with pigments, dyes, or other ingredients to create colored powders with varying degrees of pearlescence. If you want a matte powder or a very intense color, steer clear of micas and stick to the pure pigments.

OPAQUE WHITENING AGENTS such as titanium dioxide, kaolin, and zinc oxide are added to give products more coverage. Because they are generally white or off-white, these powders are also used to alter the tint of a final product.

All of these color additives are readily available for sale online through the vendors listed in the resources (page 251), but choosing among the many options can be daunting. The quality of powder and intensity of color can vary dramatically depending on the source. In addition, some retailers sell color additives coated with waxes, amino acids, or other minerals — any of which can change how the base ingredient looks and interacts with other ingredients in your recipes. These surface treatments should be clearly labeled in any product catalog, so you can avoid them if you like. Matching specific pigments and micas can be a more difficult chore. The following chart identifies each mica and pigment I used to create the recipes in this book. Many are offered through multiple websites, though often they are given different names by different vendors. A list of common names for each color is available in the Mica and Pigment Substitutions Made Easy chart (page 234).

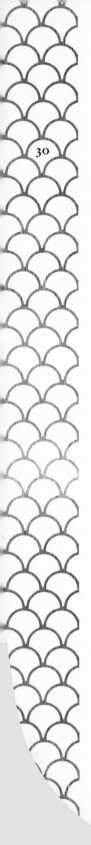

MICAS IN MY RECIPES

BRIGHT RED

BURGUNDY

GLIMMERING
BROWN BLUE

GLIMMERING
WHITE

METALLIC
GOLD

METALLIC
OLIVE

METALLIC ORANGE

MUTED GOLD

MUTED SILVER

NUDE SILVER

PALE YELLOW GREEN

PEACH GOLD

PINK BLUE

SALMON

SATIN BEIGE

SATIN BLACK

SATIN BRONZE

SATIN BROWN
BLUE

SATIN COPPER

SATIN GOLD

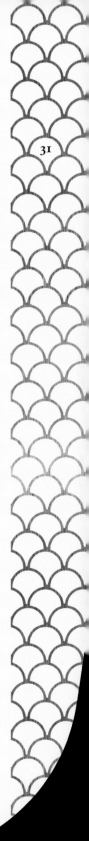

SATIN SIENNA

SATIN WHITE

SILVER GOLD

SMOKY BLUE

SMOKY GOLD

SMOKY GREEN

WHITE GOLD

PIGMENTS IN MY RECIPES

BLACK IRON
OXIDE

CHROMIUM
OXIDE GREEN

HYDRATED CHROMIUM
OXIDE GREEN

MANGANESE
VIOLET

RED IRON
OXIDE

TITANIUM
DIOXIDE

ULTRAMARINE
BLUE

ULTRAMARINE
PINK

ULTRAMARINE
VIOLET

YELLOW IRON
OXIDE

One of the main reasons to make your own cosmetics is to get exactly the color you want. Because color is so crucial, do your homework before you purchase pigments and micas to use in your recipes! This will ensure that you get exactly what you want and need. Regardless of what kind of color additives you decide to use, first make a base for each type of makeup you want. Then you can play around with creating colors by adding pigments, micas, and opaque whitening agents.

CREATING YOUR OWN COLORS

Once you have tried the recipes in this book, you will want to experiment with customizing recipes. Add your unique twist on things to create products that are completely yours. Start mixing your own colors by adding one pigment at a time so that you can see the effect after each addition. This will help you truly understand how colors work together. It is also smart to add the smallest amount of pigment that you can initially, and then incorporate more if needed. I like to put in only half of the pigment or mica quantity that a recipe calls for and see if I like

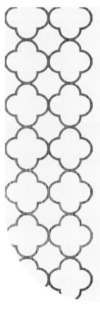

BEAUTY SPOT
FROM PIGMENT TO PRODUCT

For foundations, use **titanium dioxide, iron oxides, and ultramarine blue** to create a perfect match for your skin.

For blush and lip colors, you will mostly use **red iron oxide** and **manganese violet.**

For eye shadows and eyeliners, there are lots of color options! You can use any **ultramarines, iron oxides,** or **manganese violet.**

For highlighters, use micas with just a bit of color, such as **satin gold,** instead of matte pigments.

the color or if I should add more. It is easier to add more color than to adjust the rest of the recipe to counterbalance too much color.

Get accustomed to recording your recipes in a notebook, even when you are just experimenting. Keep track of measurements, mixing times, and the results of your recipe. You never know when you'll stumble on a formula you want to repeat! While you're at it, label your swatches and batches of your products. This helps you keep track of shades you want to make again.

Customizing Recipes for Your Skin

As you experiment with creating your own recipes, keep in mind that you will be applying makeup over skin, which already has its own natural tones. Your makeup should work well with your skin shade and skin undertone.

SKIN SHADE refers to how light or dark a person's skin is. It is relatively easy to create mineral cosmetics for light skin, as some of the primary ingredients are white and blend easily into fair skin. Making cosmetics for darker skin requires more forethought to avoid an ashen look. If you are adding color and creating a base for medium skin shades, substitute titanium oxide for zinc oxide. For dark skin shades, eliminate all titanium dioxide and zinc and use iron oxides instead. This will help you achieve coverage and the right color, without appearing ashy.

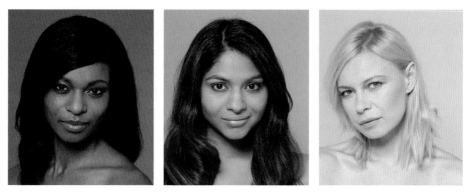

*Mixing your own foundation gives you the power to create a perfect match,
no matter how dark or light your skin is.*

SKIN UNDERTONE refers to the color that shines through from beneath a person's skin. It can be warm, neutral, or cool. To create cosmetics for warm undertones, use yellow or golden pigments. Makeup for cool undertones should incorporate blue and cool red pigments. And for those with neutral undertones, you can use warm or cool colors or a mixture.

WHAT COLOR IS YOUR SKIN UNDERTONE?

Your skin color, hair color, and eye color are all pretty obvious. But how do you know what your skin *undertone* is? Answering these questions should help.

WHAT COLOR ARE YOUR VEINS? Look at the veins on the inside of your wrist. If they appear bluish or purple, you have cool undertones. Green veins mean you have warm undertones. If you have a hard time determining whether your veins are green or blue, you have some neutral undertones.

HOW DOES YOUR FACE LOOK NEXT TO A CLEAN WHITE SHEET OF PAPER OR WRAPPED IN A WHITE TOWEL? To get accurate results, make sure you try this in natural light with a makeup-free face! If your face has a bluish shadow, your undertones are cool. Hints of yellow suggest warm undertones, and greenish tones mean you are neutral.

WHAT KIND OF JEWELRY DO YOU WEAR? If you tend to wear silver, you most likely have cool undertones. A preference for gold suggests warm undertones. If you look equally good in both silver and gold, your undertones are neutral.

WHAT HAPPENS WHEN YOU GO IN THE SUN? If you burn quickly, chances are your undertones are cool. If instead you tan, you likely have warm undertones.

Warm skin undertones are golden, peachy, or yellow. If you have warm undertones, your skin will appear peachy or golden, and you probably tan well. People with warm skin undertones often have blonde, strawberry blonde, medium brown, or black hair, with golden or red highlights, though redheads can have warm skin undertones, too. Their eyes tend to be light brown, medium brown, hazel, warm green, or blue. Warm-skinned people often look better wearing cream and muted earth-tone colors than they do wearing white and clear "true" colors.

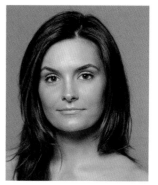

warm

Cool skin undertones are pink, red, or bluish. If you have cool undertones, your skin will appear either pink or bluish, and you probably burn more than you tan. People with cool skin undertones often have hair that is ash blonde, red, medium brown, dark brown, or coal black, with cool ashy undercurrents. Their eyes tend to be blue, green, cool green, or black brown. Cool-skinned people often look better wearing white and bright jewel-toned colors than they do wearing muted or muddy colors.

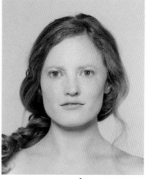

cool

Neutral skin undertones contain a combination of warm and cool coloring. People with neutral undertones can have any hair and eye color, and they wear both warm and cool colors well.

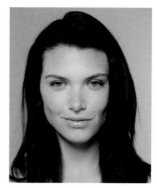

neutral

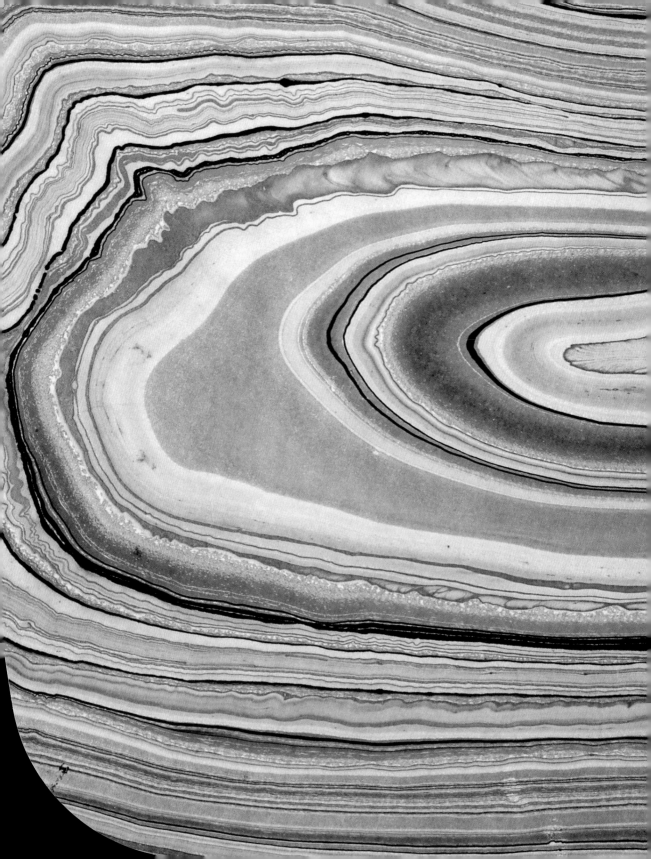

CHAPTER 3

INGREDIENTS ARE ELEMENTAL

You don't need much to change the entire world for the better. You can start with the most ordinary ingredients. You can start with the world you've got.

CATHERINE RYAN HYDE

Quality ingredients are fundamental to creating wonderful products. To select the most beneficial ingredients for your purposes, you should know a little about all the ingredients used in mineral makeup. This will also help you customize formulations and substitute ingredients. In this chapter I introduce you to the kinds of ingredients I use in my recipes and explain the considerations you should keep in mind if you decide to develop your own recipes or substitute ingredients in mine. Thorough information on each ingredient, including tips for different skin types, is available in the ingredients glossary (page 236). In addition, the Ingredients at a Glance chart (page 232) and Mica and Pigment Substitutions Made Easy chart (page 234) are quick references as you begin experimenting with recipes.

PRODUCED FOR PURITY

Some people argue that the ingredients used to create mineral makeup are not natural because they are formulated in a laboratory rather than mined directly from the earth. But that doesn't mean the ingredients are not pure. In fact, the opposite is true: producing these powders in a lab ensures that they are free from impurities that could irritate your skin or alter the color of your product. High-quality mineral makeup ingredients are chemically identical to minerals found in nature.

Producing these powders in a lab ensures that they are free from impurities that could irritate your skin or alter the color of your product.

To better understand this principle, consider a chemical compound that most everyone is familiar with: water. It's made up of two hydrogen atoms and one oxygen atom. In a laboratory, if you mix hydrogen in its gas form with oxygen in its gas form, a chemical reaction will split apart the individual molecules that make up each gas. The resulting separated atoms will rejoin to create new atoms. When one of the oxygen atoms joins with two of the hydrogen atoms, a molecule of water is created. Even though this water was created in a lab, it is still water. It is safe to drink, and you can use it to clean. The same principle is true for mineral makeup ingredients such as sericite, iron oxide, and zinc oxide. Cosmetic-grade iron oxide, for instance, is a chemical compound made from iron and oxygen. Although these mineral ingredients are technically synthetic because they have been configured and refined in a lab, they are also pure, and repeated studies have proved that they are safe.

There are other man-made ingredients, however, that are not chemically identical to mineral elements. The most common ones found in store-bought cosmetics are FD&C dyes — those approved by the U.S. Food and Drug Administration for use in food, drugs, and cosmetics. These synthetic pigments are derived from coal tar, a petroleum by-product. Some people like to use these brightly colored dyes, which are regulated by the FDA, because they result in vibrant cosmetics. None of the recipes in this book use FD&C dyes, because I prefer using pure mineral ingredients.

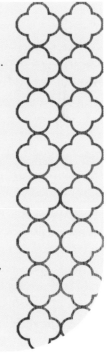

BEAUTY SPOT
GOT VEGAN?

When you create your own cosmetics, you have the power to customize your mixes to reflect your personal preferences and beliefs. Perhaps you want to use only vegan ingredients. If so, you should avoid beeswax, silk powder, micas colored with carmine, and some allantoin, magnesium myristate, magnesium stearate, and zinc stearate formulations. The ingredients glossary (page 236) and the Ingredients at a Glance chart (page 232) provide more information on which ingredients used in this book are vegan. Because some ingredients have both vegan and non-vegan options and some color additives are not vegan, always verify the composition of what you're purchasing with your vendor if you don't want anything containing animal by-products.

PROPERTIES OF INGREDIENTS

Each ingredient used in mineral makeup is unique and has a variety of properties. Before using any ingredient in a recipe, familiarize yourself with it thoroughly. Make sure you know what it looks like, how it feels, how it performs, and if you can substitute it for another ingredient.

You can usually buy inexpensive samples of the ingredients you want to try before committing to a larger size. Rub each ingredient between your hands and apply it to your jawline. Note the feel, color, and coverage. Do you like how it applies? Notice its finish: is it dewy, matte, sheer, or opaque? Try rubbing it off to test whether it smears or stays put. Play around with each ingredient until you understand how it feels, how it performs, and how its unique qualities come into play.

In addition, many individual ingredients are available with different surface treatments, or coatings, designed to improve the performance and/or feel of the base ingredient. As you select your samples, pay attention to which surface treatments, if any, you want to add, since these can dramatically change the look, feel, and effect of the final products you make.

Where Does It Come From?

This book is about mineral makeup, and I have already described the many benefits of using pure mineral ingredients. While I prefer to create all-mineral products, I find plant-based ingredients, or *botanicals,* to be helpful in some recipes and choose to include them as I see a need. Many botanicals, including cornstarch, arrowroot powder, and tapioca starch, are less expensive than mineral ingredients and can offer nondrying oil control. Some are also soothing and healing to the skin. The downside of using plant-based powders is that, unlike pure minerals, they are not inert, which means they can harbor bacteria and go bad. This is most likely to happen if these powders come into contact with moisture. To prolong the shelf life of raw botanical powders and the recipes that include them, always store your products in a cool, dry place.

INGREDIENT CATEGORIES

Each of these six categories describes certain ingredient properties. Understanding them will make substitutions easier. For more information on the categorization of specific ingredients, see the ingredients glossary (page 236).

ADHESIVES are the ingredients that help your makeup last all day. Adhesives provide very little slip, offering instead coverage and adhesion.

BINDERS have emollient and lubricating properties that create a creamy texture, which makes it easier to press loose powders into professional-looking compacts.

COLOR ADDITIVES give color and depth to your cosmetics. They can create bright and deeply colored products or add pastel hints to your foundations. Without color additives, your makeup would be white or colorless.

HEALING ingredients allow your makeup to be both pretty *and* purposeful. Skin-healing ingredients will soothe and nourish your skin while you wear your makeup.

OIL-ABSORBING ingredients soak up oil and sweat to help keep oily skin in check. These ingredients also keep your makeup colors true throughout the day.

SLIPS are the soft ingredients that enable makeup to apply smoothly and look sheer. They are often translucent. The more you add to your recipe, the lighter your formula will be, resulting in less coverage.

How Does It Work with Your Skin?

One of the main reasons people choose to wear mineral makeup is because the ingredients can provide real benefits to the skin, including absorbing oil, moisturizing, healing, and offering protection from the sun.

Although mineral makeup isn't specifically known for its *moisturizing* qualities, there are ingredients you can add to keep your skin moisturized. If you have dry or combination skin or are using skin-care products that contain retinoids, alpha hydroxy acids, glycolic acids, lactic acids, or any other potentially irritating, dehydrating, and epidermal-thinning ingredient, consider using in your recipes sericite and/or titanium dioxide surface-treated with oils, waxes, or silicones.

THE SKINNY ON SKIN TYPES

Knowing your skin type ensures proper care for your largest organ, resulting in a healthy canvas on which to apply your makeup. Which type you have largely depends on how much water your skin contains, the concentration of lipids in your skin, and how tolerant your skin is to external factors.

NORMAL SKIN creates and maintains a balanced amount of water and lipids, and it withstands regular variations in weather, inside temperature, and other external factors.

DRY SKIN loses moisture when its outer layer is damaged or lost. Often this is the result of extreme or prolonged exposure to sun, wind, or cold temperatures. Genetics and hormones also influence the likelihood of having dry skin, and chemicals in many beauty products can dry out the skin, too.

With the exception of surface treatments and pressed compacts, powdered mineral makeup should not contain oils or waxes, a fact that helps reduce the potential for acne and clogged pores. If you tend to have oily skin, there are a few *oil-absorbing* ingredients you can add to your makeup to absorb excess oil and minimize shine. Kaolin, silica, and calcium carbonate minimize shiny skin and help create a flawless matte look. Conveniently, these ingredients also keep your makeup colors true throughout the day. Even people with very oily skin should use these powders only in small amounts, though, to prevent overdrying. Those with dry skin should not use these powders at all. Each ingredient has a recommended concentration of use — meaning what proportion of a product it comprises — which you should not exceed to avoid unintended results.

OILY SKIN contains overactive oil glands. Hormones and stress both affect how much lipid the body produces, and as a result, the level of oiliness can change daily. Certain medications and weather factors like heat and humidity also influence oil levels.

SENSITIVE SKIN can be dry or oily but is characterized by a low tolerance to external factors. This can result in itchy or blotchy patches, and people with sensitive skin tend to flush and burn easily. Possible triggers include food, weather, and skin-care products.

In addition to these main skin types, many people have combination skin, with either oily or dry areas on the forehead, nose, and chin and other skin types elsewhere.

Finally, it is important to note that your skin type will likely change over time. Human skin often loses moisture over the years, becoming thinner and drier. Pay attention to your skin and give it what it needs — today and beyond.

Kaolin, silica, and calcium carbonate minimize shiny skin and help create a flawless matte look.

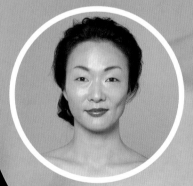

Akiko is wearing

EYES: Bambi shadow; Raven eyebrow powder

LIPS: Ruby Red

FACE: Cake foundation; Honey bronzer; Harajuku blush; Nectar highlighter

In order to create pressed compacts, you will most likely need some kind of *binding* agent to help hold the powders together. But making your own gives you control over what kind of binder you use. Your choices include powders surface-treated with wax or powders that have their own natural binding properties, like zinc stearate. If you choose to use oil instead, you have control over how much you add to your makeup, meaning that you can use oils that do not clog pores, are minimally processed, and/or are actually beneficial to certain skin types. However, because many people wear mineral makeup specifically to let their skin breathe, some may want to stay away from binding waxes and oils altogether. If you have oily, acne-prone skin, try using loose powders and avoid the ingredients I list as binders; you will still have plenty of mineral makeup options. If you have mature, dry skin, binders might be the moisturizing ingredient you need. Always consider your skin type when formulating.

Regardless of whether your skin is oily or dry, there are a handful of powerful ingredients that aid in *healing*, such as zinc, allantoin, and cornstarch. You can add these healing ingredients to any recipe to help treat sensitive skin, acne, psoriasis, eczema, and other skin conditions.

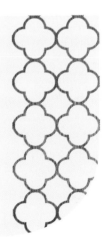

BEAUTY SPOT
SUN PROTECTION FACTOR (SPF)

Some ingredients — including titanium dioxide, zinc oxide, allantoin, kaolin, silk powder, and zinc stearate — provide some sun protection. Without going through a costly review by the Food and Drug Administration, though, you cannot legally assign a sun protection factor, or SPF, number to your product. You can, however, say that your product "offers some sun protection."

How Does It Look?

Mineral makeup generally provides fairly heavy *coverage*, meaning it camouflages your skin well. When mixing up recipes, if you want to increase the coverage, add matte pigment and decrease the proportion of sericite. Create a more sheer coverage by adding translucent powders such as sericite.

The adhesion and slip of an ingredient also influence the final product's coverage. *Adhesion* refers to how well an ingredient sticks to the skin. Usually the more adhesion the ingredient has, the more opaque it is and the greater coverage it provides. *Slip* refers to how well an ingredient glides over your skin. Ingredients with a lot of slip also make the finished products more sheer. Both adhesion and slip are important properties, as one helps your makeup resist smudging and the other helps it apply evenly. You definitely want a good balance between the two. Ingredients with too much adhesion create heavy powders that drag and result in a patchy application. Too much slip results in makeup that won't stay in place and doesn't offer much coverage.

Regardless of your desired coverage, the ingredients you use can create very different looks for your finished products. A *matte* finish helps hide acne, uneven skin color or texture, and other perceived skin "flaws," while a *lustrous* finish provides a youthful, pearlescent glow that draws attention to the surface of the skin. Lustrous ingredients tend to be fillers, or "extra" ingredients added to give the finished product a certain quality, such as binding or shine.

The finish an ingredient offers is influenced by its *particle size*, or the length of the elements that comprise it. In cosmetics, the standard unit of measurement is a micron, which equals one thousandth of a millimeter, or about 0.000039 inch. A lower particle size results in less light reflected from the makeup, creating a matte finish with more coverage. A higher particle size results in more luster and less coverage.

Some powders come with the option of either micronized particles or nano-particles. Micronized particles are usually between 0.1 micron and 100 microns, while nanoparticles are even smaller. Because these smallest particles result in an extremely sheer powder, nanoparticles are often used in sunscreens; they allow you to lather on a lot of lotion without taking on an opaque white cast. However, some studies show that nanoparticles can enter the skin, possibly causing health problems. Because testing hasn't been done on the long-term effects of nano-particle powders, I recommend sticking with the higher-micron powders, as they are not believed to enter the skin.

COLOR EFFECT	PARTICLE SIZE
Low luster and good hiding power	15 microns or less
Silky luster and strong hiding power	2–25 microns
Pearl luster and medium hiding power	10–60 microns
Shimmering luster and low hiding power	10–125 microns
Sparkling luster and transparent	20–150 microns
Glittering luster and very transparent	45–500 microns

A micron, or micrometer, equals one thousandth of a millimeter, or about 0.000039 inch.
Source: cosmeticpigments.com

A few ingredients contain *light-scattering particles*, which create a soft focus similar to the dreamlike glow that old-time cinematographers used to give the female beauties in their films. In photography the image is blurred by altering how the light rays move through the sphere of a lens, and the same basic principle is used in cosmetics to smooth the appearance of fine lines. Wrinkles are crevices, and like all narrow openings, light gets trapped in them. The contrast between the shaded lines and the rest of the face is what attracts the eye. Light-scattering particles minimize the amount of light the skin absorbs and transmit the majority of the remaining light diffusely. By giving the eye more rays of light to take in simultaneously, the contrast between the wrinkle and the rest of the face is diminished, giving the appearance of smoother skin.

MICA AND SERICITE

Sericite is a type of mica that is widely used as one of the primary ingredients in mineral makeup. Cosmetic-grade *sericite mica* is a finely ground off-white powder with a small amount of luster. In the world of mineral makeup, *mica* — not preceded by *sericite* — generally refers to the wide range of opalescent colors that are added to eye shadows, highlighters, lip gloss, or anything else that sparkles. Although mica occurs in nature in shades ranging from white to green, mica colorants used in makeup are created by treating fine mica flakes with nature-identical iron oxides and ultramarines as well as with synthetic dyes and carmine. When creating the recipes for this book, I used only micas made with iron oxides, ultramarines, and carmine; none contain synthetic dyes.

To avoid confusion, in this book I use the term *sericite* to refer to the white powder that is the primary ingredient in my makeup bases. I reserve *mica* for reference to pearlescent color additives.

Mica offers a wide range of opalescent colors that sparkle.

Janel is wearing

EYES: Buttercream and Fairy Floss shadows; Sun-Kissed eyeliner

FACE: Eggnog foundation; Honey bronzer; Vamp blush; Flurries highlighter

LIPS: Basic Lip Gloss mixed with burgundy mica

SAFE USE

Always put safety first, and protect yourself and others! Never use ingredients that are contaminated or have expired, and always use makeup as intended.

While micas, oxides, and other powders are sold as supplies in many types of stores — including automotive, pottery, soap making, painting, and other arts and crafts — these are not cosmetic-grade pigments. Do not use them interchangeably with your makeup ingredients! In addition, never use crayons, spices, colored pencils, chalk, activated charcoal, fruit, food coloring, or glitter to color your makeup. None of these common items are approved by the FDA for use on your skin. You should also avoid using in your makeup the common food-grade versions of ingredients such as arrowroot powder and tapioca starch. The powders that you find in the grocery store usually have a higher micron size than their cosmetic counterparts, may result in a grainy texture, and might contain traces of other ingredients. Any powder used in cosmetic formulations should be no larger than 150 microns.

Some cosmetic-grade pigments and ingredients should be used only for certain kinds of products that are used only on specific parts of the body. For example, the FDA has not approved chromium oxide green, ultramarine, and ferric ferrocyanide for use in lip products. Other ingredients are restricted to a certain percentage of the ingredients in a product. For detailed information about restrictions associated with specific ingredients, visit the ingredients glossary (page 236). For a complete current list of approved colorants and their restrictions, refer to the FDA website, www.fda.gov. Also, remember that every country has unique health guidelines, so what is restricted in one country might be allowed in another. If you will be selling your products, be sure to obey the regulations in the country where you will market them.

Protecting Your Lungs

Frequently inhaling large quantities loose particles can harm your respiratory system, but making mineral makeup does not have to be a dangerous project. Whenever you mix powders, wear a face mask to protect yourself from breathing them in. This is especially important if you are using a blender or other mechanical grinder, since mixing powders at a high speed creates a dust cloud. As an added precaution, let the mixture settle before opening the grinder.

In addition, when you measure powders or move them from one container to another, scoop them carefully with a spoon or cup. Never dump the powder directly from its original container as this can also create a cloud of dust. Finally, once you have finished mixing your recipes, always apply your makeup as directed, without stirring up an excess of loose powders. This is especially true for titanium dioxide.

Allergic Reactions and Emergencies

Each ingredient you buy should have a batch number and a material safety data sheet, or MSDS. The FDA requires that these documents include storage information for the ingredient and what to do in case of a fire or ingestion. The MSDS should also specify any restrictions on the ingredient. For products that contain multiple ingredients — such as colored mica or a prepared base or color blend for cosmetics — the sheet should include a complete contents list. You should be able to view this information readily on the supplier's website, or you can request a copy from the seller. Store these sheets in a secure place, and keep track of the safety information for each ingredient. If there is ever an emergency — including ingestion of large quantities of powders — follow the directions on the safety sheet and/or call poison control.

Substitutions

Always consider your options. Almost every ingredient in the recipes that follow can be easily replaced by a substitute. If you would prefer to avoid a certain ingredient, or want to use something you have on hand, check out the Ingredients at a Glance chart (page 232). Before you substitute for anything, make sure you understand what purpose the original ingredient serves in the recipe, and find an alternative from the same property category.

Avoiding Ingredients

The ingredients glossary (page 236) includes ingredients typically used for making mineral makeup, even if they are not in any of my recipes. Some I recommend avoiding altogether, but I included them so you could learn more about some of the common mineral makeup ingredients. Make the choice for yourself whether to incorporate them in your cosmetics.

Two controversial ingredients in particular that are found in many commercial cosmetics are bismuth and talc. *Bismuth oxychloride*, sometimes called synthetic pearl, is a fine white powder that adheres well to the skin and provides a pearly, high-luster look. Its crystalline structure can irritate the pores, especially when it is used as the main ingredient. I do not recommend using this ingredient, especially if you have sensitive skin, acne, or any other skin conditions, as it is a known irritant that makes skin itch and worsens skin irritation. *Talc* is the primary ingredient in talcum powder, and there is a lot of controversy surrounding it. Some say it clogs pores, while others claim talcum powder used around the genitals can cause ovarian cancer. Given all the negative associations with talc, I stay away from it. There are many safe ingredients that give your cosmetic bases the same adhesion and soft feel as talc, without any of the risks.

FDA Regulations

Even if you do not plan to sell your cosmetics, it is a good idea to comply with government safety rules and regulations for ingredient use. Likewise, if you ever have a question about the safety of an ingredient, look it up!

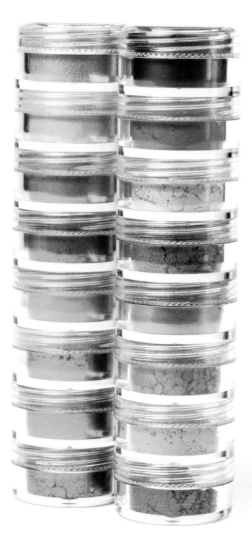

The Food and Drug Administration's website, www.FDA.gov, has an entire section on cosmetics, with detailed information on ingredients and contaminants. If you live outside the United States, check your government's regulatory agency. Chances are there will be helpful information online.

SUPPLIERS

All of the ingredients listed in this book are readily available online. But before you purchase anything, it's wise to know what you're getting. Retailers should be able to provide you with basic information about the ingredients, along with detailed material safety data sheets.

When buying from a retailer for the first time, start with small quantities. That way you can test the quality of both the ingredients and the customer service. If the seller doesn't seem to know about the ingredients or makeup in general, or is reluctant to answer your questions, try another store. To ensure that you are getting safe ingredients, familiarize yourself with FDA cosmetic regulations. This will help you be aware if any suppliers are not complying with federal regulations or are supplying you with unsafe ingredients.

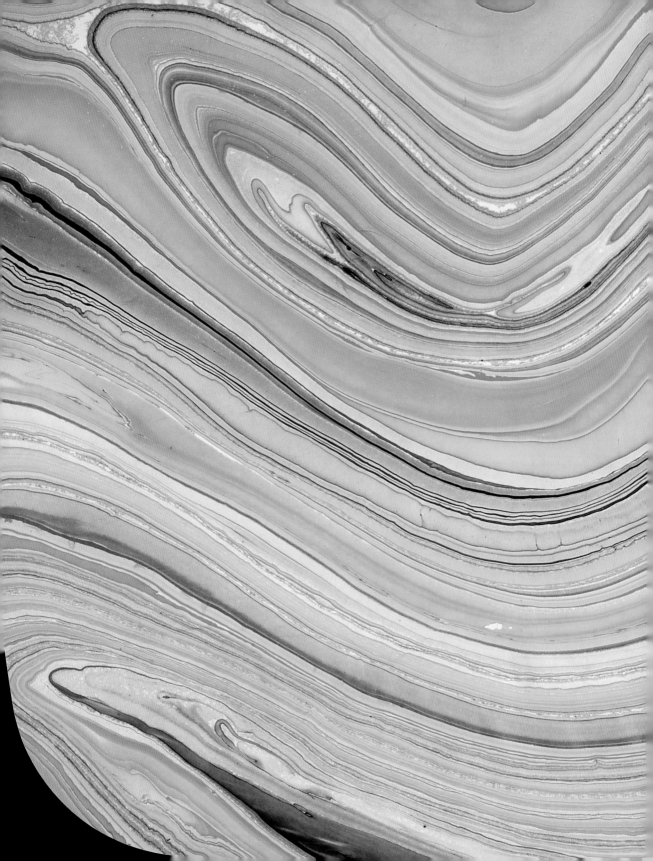

CHAPTER 4

CHOOSING EQUIPMENT AND TOOLS

This world is but a canvas to our imagination.

HENRY DAVID THOREAU

The equipment you select to make your mineral makeup is just as important as the ingredients themselves. In this chapter I introduce you to the tools of the trade, recommending certain items that will streamline your makeup making and give your products a clean, professional look. If you're itching to get going but don't have the tools I recommend, don't worry! For the most part, you can start with just a bowl and a spoon.

Even the full list of tools I recommend mostly contains items that can be found at your local grocery store or online. Only use new equipment that has *never* prepared food and will never be used for anything other than creating makeup. Equipment that has been employed for anything else can spread bacteria and contaminate your makeup.

These basic tools will help you whip up products faster and with less mess, and they will give your makeup a professional finish.

▸ Mini measuring spoons, including tad, dash, pinch, smidgen, and drop (available for purchase at most kitchen supply stores)

▸ Battery-operated herb or tobacco grinder (or food processor, mini blender, or coffee grinder) to mix matte powders

▸ Face mask to protect your lungs

▸ Small cups (or shot glasses, bowls, or candle votives) to mix your makeup

▸ Metal spoon or whisk to mix powders with liquids

▸ New packaging, such as pans, compacts, jars, makeup palettes, bottles, or tubes, for your chosen project

▸ Cleanup material, such as baby wipes, rags, or paper towels

MEASURING TOOLS

To keep your recipes and colors consistent, always measure out your ingredients. Heatproof measuring cups allow you to measure and then heat liquid lip-product ingredients in the same container, saving time. When working with powders, mini measuring spoons are handy, but because the density of micas and powders can vary from color to color, measuring ingredients by weight with a pocket scale

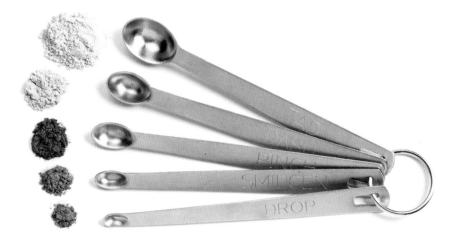

is more precise and will result in more consistent products. Because the recipes in
this book are intended for beginners, I list measuring spoon amounts rather than
weights. As you become more comfortable with the process and want to duplicate
specific colors, consider investing in an accurate scale that measures in grams.

OPTIONAL TOOLS

Once you get more advanced, you can splurge on some
or all of this equipment.

- » **New paintbrush**, makeup brush, drafting
  brush, or scraper for cleaning your work surface
  and mixing cups
- » **Tamping tool**, such as a clean, sanded wooden
  dowel or metal rod, to press your powders
- » **Textured surfaces**, including fabrics — such
  as denim, corduroy, or lace — or stamps, to make
  imprints and designs on your pressed powders
- » **Metal flavor injector**, such as what
  you would use to inject meat with butter, or
  5-milliliter syringes, to fill lip gloss containers
- » **Bead organizers** or jars to store pigments,
  micas, and powders
- » **Mini pocket scale** with units smaller than
  grams to measure ingredients more accurately
- » **Lab journal**, notebook, or binder to keep
  track of swatches, samples, recipes, and
  inspiration
- » **Apron** to protect your clothing
- » **Surface covering**, such as waxed paper,
  cutting board, place mat, mirror, or silicone mat

MIXING TOOLS

Electric mixing tools are important for creating flawless, streak-free products. Micas can be blended by hand, but if you plan on making any matte makeup, a motorized blender is a must. (See page 65 for an example.) This does not have to be an expensive undertaking. You can purchase a small battery-operated herb or tobacco grinder online for as little as $10.

When mixing powders into liquids, any kind of stirrer will do. I prefer a metal spatula or small metal whisk because they are easy to clean and disinfect. If you decide to use wooden popsicle sticks or coffee stirrers, be sure to use a clean new one each time to avoid bacterial contamination and mixing colors. You will also need to make sure that no wood splinters break off into your product.

If you plan on making both liquid and powder products, get separate measuring tools, mixing tools, and machines for each to avoid spreading bacteria.

PACKAGING

Always package your makeup in clean containers to keep your cosmetics free from bacteria. Make sure your packaging is fully sanitized and dry before starting your project.

Most of the jars you will use for mineral makeup come in standard sizes: 3, 5, 10, 20, and 30 grams. These numbers refer to how much water the jar can hold. A 5-gram jar, for instance, can hold 5 grams of water. Because water has a different density than powder — and each mineral makeup powder you mix will likely have its own unique density — the figures associated with the jar sizes are not the same as the amount of makeup the jar will hold. The following table is a general guide for how much mineral makeup each jar should contain.

JAR SIZE	HOLDS THIS AMOUNT OF MAKEUP
5 grams	1.25–1.5 grams
10 grams	2.5–3 grams
20 grams	5–6 grams
30 grams	7.5–9 grams

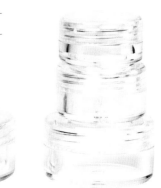

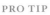

PRO TIP

HOW LONG WILL IT LAST?

You might be wondering how long an amount of makeup will last before it's all gone. This varies widely, depending on the specific product, how much you use, and your application method. Here is a rough estimate of what to expect.

PRODUCT	JAR SIZE	WILL LAST YOU
Eye shadow	3 grams	1 month
	5 grams	2–3 months
	10 grams	6 months
Foundation	10 grams	4–6 months
	20 grams	9–12 months
	30 grams	12–18 months

In addition to the containers themselves, these extra items will come in handy but are optional.

MAGNETS OR GLUE will secure your pressed palettes or compacts.

SHRINK BANDS give a professional appearance to your finished products. If you plan to sell your cosmetics, these will assure customers that their makeup product has not been tampered with.

MINI RESEALABLE PLASTIC BAGS from the bead section of a craft store are the perfect size for storing extra pigments and samples.

CIRCULAR LABELS are handy for naming and dating your products.

PRESSING TOOLS

If you want to press any of your eye shadows, be sure to get a pressing tool just barely smaller than the pan into which you are pressing. There are many options available. A sanitized coin, silicone mat, or pressing tile will get the job done, but I prefer to use a tamping tool because it is easier to grip and increases the force of your pressing. You can make your own by affixing a handle or knob to a plastic tile.

While you are pressing your powders, you can give them a decorative embossed finish by placing any clean textured surface over the top of your product and under your pressing tool. At most fabric stores, you can purchase remnants or

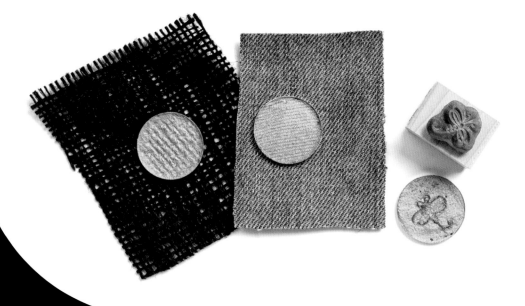

2-inch swatches very inexpensively. Those with a loose, thick weave generally work better than tightly woven fabric. Pick up a few different fabrics or stamps and try them out to see which design you like best in your finished makeup.

FILLING TOOLS

Most mineral makeup is in a dry, powdered form and can be easily transferred from your mixing container to your product container. For the few liquid products you may create — such as lip gloss — you will need an efficient way to get the final form into a container. While disposable syringes are nice for filling small containers and removing excess liquid from a lip gloss tube, metal flavor injectors help large lip gloss batches go more quickly. The reusable injector will also save you money in the long run. I have one injector for each type of product I make, plus I keep a few plastic syringes on hand for especially messy projects.

STORAGE AND LABELING

It is your responsibility to ensure the safety of your products, regardless of whether you decide to sell them. Store your finished products in a cool, dark, dry place, off the floor. Be sure to note the creation date and ingredients on the container of any cosmetics you make.

While you don't have to purchase special storage or organization equipment, you may find it easier to keep track of your ingredients with some compartmentalized containers. Most of the ingredients you buy will come in plastic bags, which can easily rip and spill. Transferring your micas, pigments, and other powders to jars will help protect your ingredients. Plastic containers designed to organize beads are both perfect for this use and readily available at most craft stores.

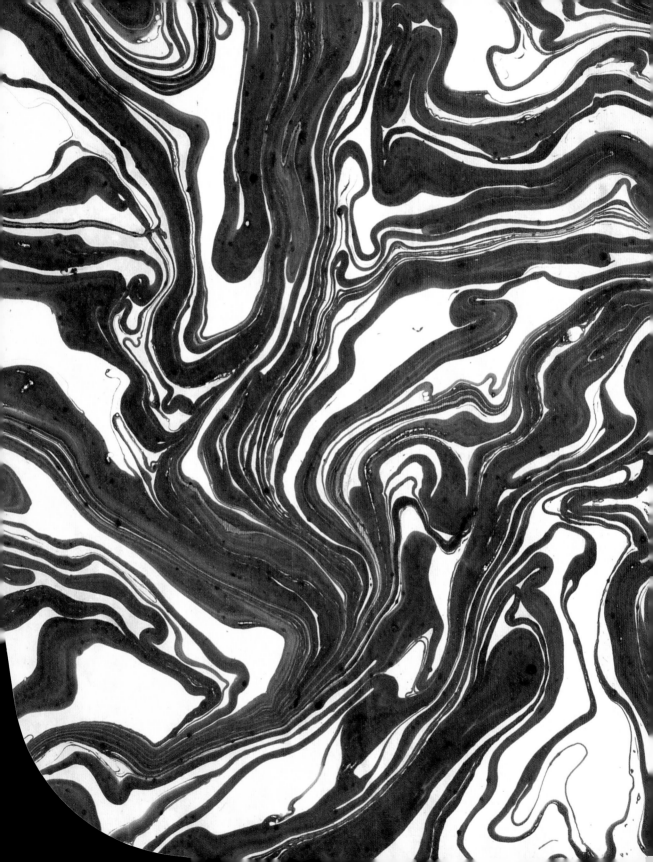

CHAPTER 5

MAKING MAKEUP, STEP BY STEP

When a creature begins to emerge from its chrysalis there is a point at which it is neither one thing nor the other, not quite grown into a new identity nor rid of the old. . . . It is that long still moment of waiting that fascinates me utterly. The suspense of waiting for beauty to unfurl.

MEG ROSOFF

In this chapter, you will learn how to mix multiple powders, mix powders into liquids, fill containers, and press compacts. Before starting on a cosmetics project, it is a good idea to practice the techniques outlined here using inexpensive ingredients to avoid waste.

My instructions and tips should help streamline your makeup-making process. But don't worry if you make a mess! I do all the time. Just be prepared to clean up your workspace and yourself when you're done.

PREPARING YOUR WORKSPACE

Your first step in making cosmetics is to set up a sanitary workspace. This is key to protecting yourself and others by preventing the spread of germs into your makeup. Proper ventilation, such as an exhaust fan or air purifier or a box fan pointed away from your workspace, helps keep small particles from entering your lungs. In addition, always wear a face mask when working with any powdered ingredient to protect your lungs from fine particles.

Follow these steps to ensure that you don't forget anything.

- Review the recipe and collect all the tools, ingredients, and packaging you will use.
- Wash each tool and piece of equipment — including the packaging you will put your finished products into — with hot water and a gentle dish detergent. Rinse well, making sure there's no residue, and let each item air-dry.
- Spray each fully dry tool with a sanitizer such as rubbing (isopropyl) alcohol, then let air-dry before using.
- Clear off your work surface, sanitize it with rubbing alcohol, and set up your surface covering, if you're using one.
- Pull back your hair, wash your hands, and put on a face mask and an apron. If you are making makeup for sale, wear clean latex or nitrile gloves to keep your products free of germs.

MIXING POWDERS

Nearly all the ingredients in my recipes come in powder form, and with the exception of lip balm, lip gloss, and mixing medium, all the recipes in this book make powdered products. Combining multiple powders is not complicated, but matte pigments and lustrous micas do require different mixing methods to preserve their trademark characteristics.

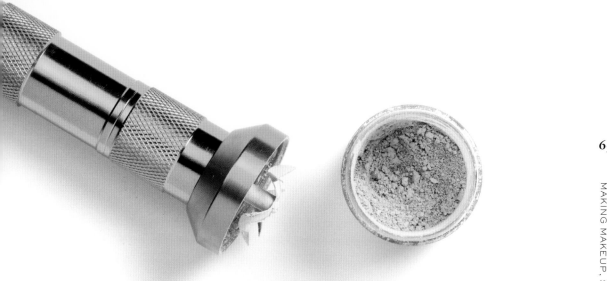

How to Mix Matte Powders

Matte powders and pigments such as iron oxides and ultramarines are very dense and should always be mixed mechanically. You can use a mini blender or a small battery-operated herb or tobacco grinder. All of these tools will help you create a finer powder and streak-free color. Hand-mixing matte pigments will result in streaks of color, which can ruin the makeup application.

Recipes in this book that need to be electrically mixed include makeup base, matte eye shadows, matte eyeliner, matte eyebrow powder, foundation bases, foundation, concealer, color correctors, finishing powder, matte blush, and matte bronzer.

PRO TIP
TROUBLESHOOTING WHEN MIXING POWDERS

PROBLEM	SOLUTION
Too sheer	Add titanium dioxide or pigments.
Too heavy	Add sericite.
Streaky	Mix longer with an electric mixer.

How to Mix Pearlescent Powders

To mix micas and other pearlescent powders into matte powder, makeup base, or sheer powder like arrowroot, cornstarch, or tapioca starch, you'll want to work by hand to ensure that their luster isn't dulled. Mixing colored micas by machine breaks up the sparkly surface, resulting in less shine. While you are experimenting with creating your own makeup, add one mica at a time and mix after each addition. This will help you understand how every change affects the color and

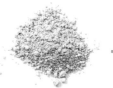 + =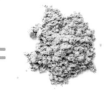

makeup base and ultramarine pink *silver gold mica*

BEAUTY SPOT
MAKING MAKEUP DOS AND DON'TS

Always
Wash your hands thoroughly.
Wear a protective face mask, clean clothing, and an apron.
Pull your hair back or wear a hat or hairnet.

Never
Eat, drink, or smoke while making cosmetics.
Leave open food containers near your makeup ingredients or finished products.
Make cosmetics when you are sick or when you have any hand wounds.
Let animals, their fur, or their dander or children come in contact with any of your supplies, equipment, or workspace.

consistency of the final product. Once you are familiar with a recipe, you can add all of the micas at once, making sure you mix thoroughly to ensure that all of the powders are distributed evenly.

You can use any of the following mixing methods for recipes with mica, including shimmery eye shadow, shimmery eyeliner, highlighter, shimmery blush, and shimmery bronzer.

MIXING IN A JAR

1. Measure your first ingredient and place it in the jar.
2. Measure your next ingredient and add it to the jar. Attach the jar's lid.
3. Shake until fully mixed.
4. Repeat with each ingredient until all the powders are fully mixed.

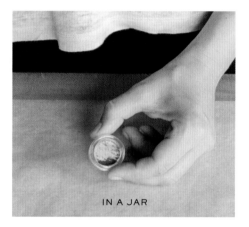

IN A JAR

MIXING IN A CUP

1. Measure your first ingredient and place it in the cup.
2. Measure your next ingredient and add it to the cup.
3. With your stirring tool, mix in circular motions until fully blended.
4. Repeat with each ingredient until all the powders are fully mixed.

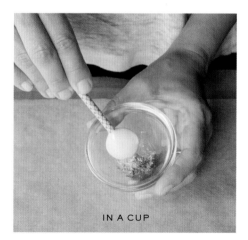

IN A CUP

MIXING IN A RESEALABLE PLASTIC BAG

1. Measure your first ingredient and place it in the plastic bag.
2. Measure your next ingredient and add it to the bag. Seal the bag.
3. Using your hands, massage the two ingredients thoroughly for a few seconds, until blended.
4. Repeat until all the ingredients have been added.

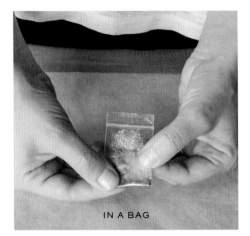

IN A BAG

MIXING LIQUIDS

You will rarely work with liquids because mineral makeup tends to be in powder form. Lip gloss and lip balm bases are the only liquid products I include in this book. Complete instructions for mixing up those products are in the Recipes for the Lips section, which begins on page 182.

You will also mix liquids with mineral powders to make pressed powders, colored lip balm, or colored lip gloss. For pressed powders, you will add small amounts of a binder and rubbing alcohol to your completed powder products, stirring until you have the consistency of wet sand. Complete directions for pressing powders begin on page 72. If you want to add color to your lip products, you can either use powdered pigments and colored mica or buy predispersed lip colorants. With the pigment already mixed into a small amount of castor oil, these predispersed products can help you avoid unwanted marbling and make a more uniformly colored lip gloss. More information about adding colors to lip products is on page 189.

FILLING CONTAINERS

Because most mineral makeup comes in the form of loose powders, filling your cosmetic containers is fairly easy, but there are a couple things to keep in mind.

When filling jars or plastic bags with powders, it is best to slowly scoop out and place the powder instead of pouring it. Dropping the powders will create a cloud of dust, which wastes product, makes a mess, and exposes you to inhaling fine powders. When filling a plastic bag, use a simple homemade paper funnel.

Pressing Powders

After mixing the pigments in with the makeup base, you can either leave your powders loose or press them into makeup jars or compacts. Pearlescent makeup presses more easily than matte powders, which are brittle and delicate. For best results when working with matte powders, leave them loose when possible. If you must press them, use small tins to minimize the cracking.

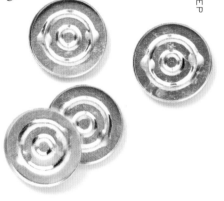

If you choose to press your mica-based powders, I recommend doing so in tin makeup pans. I find these sturdy, magnetic pans are easier to work with than aluminum pans, which are not magnetic and bend more easily. The downside to using tin is that it can rust if exposed to water. To avoid this, I clean my pans and wet my powders with 91 percent rubbing alcohol instead of the more common 70 percent solution, which has a higher water content.

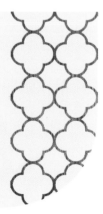

BEAUTY SPOT
PROTECT YOURSELF

Isopropyl alcohol, like all alcohol, is flammable, and the 91 percent solution is more so than the 70 percent solution. Both versions are safe to use to clean metal pans and moisten powder makeup, but be sure to keep all rubbing alcohol away from open flames and store at room temperature.

You can select from the various pan shapes and sizes available for pressed powders. Round tins are most common, but you can also find square or rectangular pans, as well as half- and quarter-circle tins, which you can piece together to form a complete circle.

To determine the size of each pan you will need, consider how much of each product you use and how often you use it. Eye shadows, eyebrow powders, and eyeliners often are pressed into 26-millimeter round metal pans, but you can opt for containers as small as 15 millimeters or as large as 36 millimeters. The most common round metal pans for blushes, bronzers, highlighters, concealers, color correctors, and foundations are 36 millimeters and 44 millimeters. A 57-millimeter round tin — the largest you can buy — fits into most single compacts.

The next step is to decide what kind of compact or palette you would like to display your makeup in. Your options are limitless; be creative! While some people purchase new palettes, others reuse old makeup containers or even make their own out of mint tins, CD or DVD cases, or other hinged boxes. As long as your container is sanitized and has a lid to keep your makeup free of dust or other contaminants, you can use practically anything as a compact.

I buy my palettes online in bulk, then line them with sticky magnetic paper so the metal pans with pressed powders stay put in the display. You can also glue your pans to the inside of the compact. Before doing so, wipe the bottom of the

Reuse your compacts by replacing old makeup tins with new, clean ones.

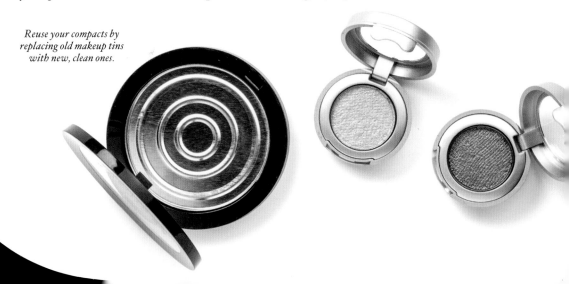

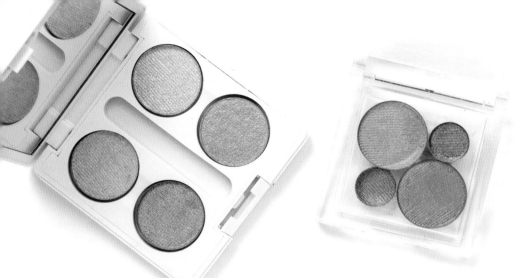

pans to remove all powder. Add a single drop of permanent adhesive craft glue or hot glue to the bottom of the pan, then place it in your container and gently press on the pan sides to secure. Lay the container down flat and let the glue set overnight.

BEAUTY SPOT
EYE SHADOW PALETTES

When applying eye shadow, you often want to blend more than one color. You can take the guesswork out of picking colors that complement each other by packaging multiple eye shadow colors together. Consider the color wheel before creating a four-tone eye shadow palette (or *quad*). Most quads include one dark, one light, and two mid-tone colors. The pale color can highlight the face and eyes; the medium colors are ideal for the eyelid color; and the dark color can create a crease, make a smoky-eye look, or serve as eyeliner. Rather than choosing random colors for these multicolor compacts, you can focus on specific color themes, such as warm, cool, neutral, monochromatic, analogous, shades, or tints.

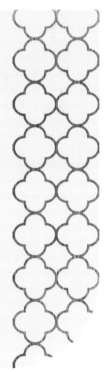

How to Press Makeup Pans

You can press lustrous loose powders into makeup pans using any tamping tool. As noted above, matte powders are extremely delicate and best left loose. Follow the directions below for a beautiful finished product.

NOTE: The quantities in these directions assume you are pressing one of my eye shadow recipes into a 26-millimeter pan. If you are making other recipes or pressing into a pan of a different size, you will need to experiment with quantities.

YOU WILL NEED

- ▶ Ingredients for the eye shadow recipe you want to press, making sure to use the Makeup Base for Pressed Powders (page 83); to fill one 26-millimeter pan, you will need to make approximately 1½ batches of the eye shadow recipe
- ▶ 1 tad fractionated coconut oil (a refined version of coconut oil often used in aromatherapy), or more as needed to reach the desired consistency
- ▶ 1 dash plus 1 pinch rubbing alcohol (preferably 91%), or more as needed to reach the desired consistency
- ▶ Your preferred mixing tools
- ▶ Tamping tool (see example at right)
- ▶ Makeup pan
- ▶ Clean fabric or stamp to create a decorative finish

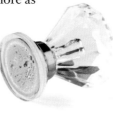

PRO TIP
KEEPING TRACK OF YOUR RECIPES

Whenever you're formulating a new recipe, write down every ingredient you use and the amount. Add your ingredients one at a time, mix after each addition, and keep track of how long you blend each round. The length of time you blend a recipe can change the color and consistency of the powder. Keeping track of the mixing time will help you replicate a color and/or texture in the future.

1. Mix together all the ingredients in the recipe you want to press, making sure there are no streaks or lumps.

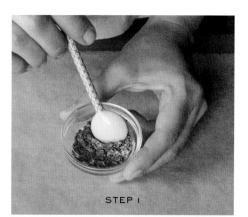

STEP 1

2. Add the fractionated coconut oil and rubbing alcohol and stir into the powders until you have the consistency of wet sand. If your mixture is not there yet, add more oil or alcohol, one drop at a time, as needed. The oil binds the powders together, while the rubbing alcohol helps to evenly distribute the oils and turns the mixture into a liquid so it can be smoothed and pressed.

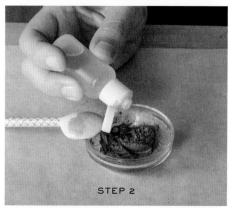

STEP 2

3. Fill the pan with the moistened powder, making sure that it is distributed evenly. Smooth out the top of the mixture.

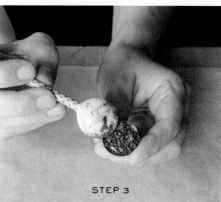

STEP 3

4. If you are using fabric to create a textured top, layer and twist it over the tamping tool to create a smooth surface.

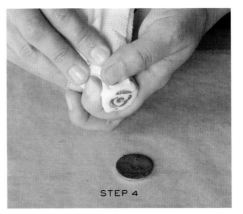

STEP 4

5. Center the tamping tool or the decorative stamp in the pan and press down firmly. Some of the liquid and color should wick through the fabric, if using. Keep pressing until most of the liquid is removed from the product.

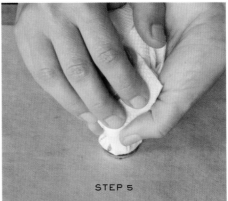

STEP 5

6. Pull the tamping tool or stamp straight up so as not to ruin the newly pressed design.
7. Let dry for 12 to 24 hours before using.

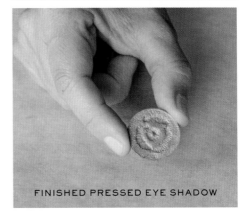

FINISHED PRESSED EYE SHADOW

PRO TIP

TROUBLESHOOTING WHEN PRESSING POWDERS

PROBLEM	SOLUTION
Too oily	Add more powder.
Too dry	Add more binder and more rubbing alcohol.
Too hard or waxy	Break up the pressed powder and add more of the finished recipe you are pressing to lower the oil-to-cosmetic ratio. Press again.
Eye shadow breaks	Thoroughly break up the powder into its loose form, then add more rubbing alcohol and binder and press again.
Marbling	Break up the pressed powder, scrape it into a resealable plastic bag, and crumble into a fine powder. Wet the powder again with rubbing alcohol, mix again, and repress. If you have already added a binder, do not add more, as that will make your pressed powder greasy.

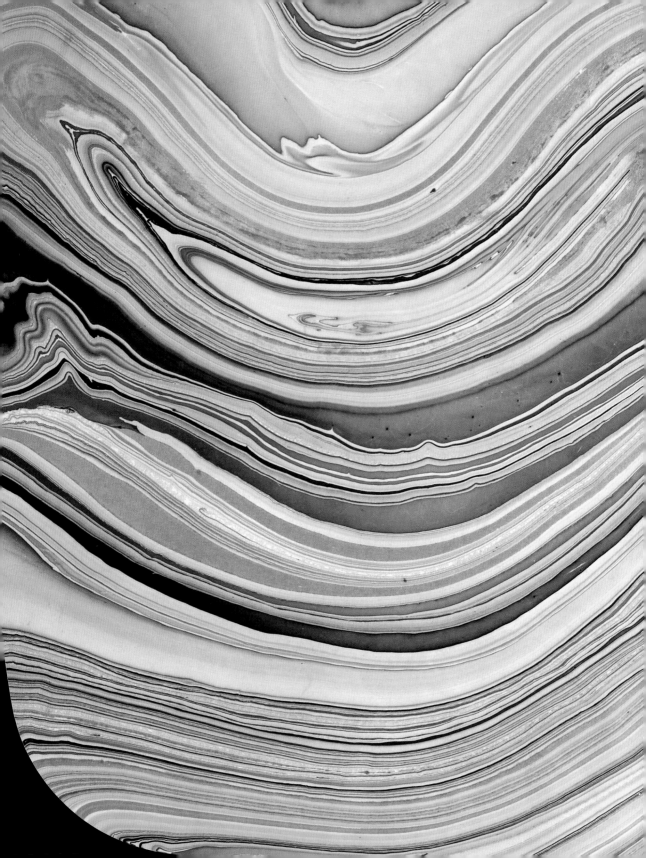

CHAPTER 6

CREATING YOUR COSMETICS

The desire to create is one of the deepest yearnings of the human soul. . . . Everyone can create. You don't need money, position, or influence in order to create something of substance or beauty.

DIETER F. UCHTDORF

You're finally ready to start making your own makeup! In this chapter I share some of my favorite recipes, starting with the least complicated and progressing to formulas that require more fine-tuning.

Eye shadows are the easiest products to whip up, as you really can never come up with a wrong color. The options are endless. Once you are comfortable with mixing eye shadows, you can experiment with other products. I recommend starting with some bronzer, eyeliner, and highlighter recipes. When you have those down, try matching your skin color, shade, and undertone while making some concealers and foundations. The more recipes you try, the greater your color knowledge and skill. I have left lip products for last because the ingredients and processes are so different from those in the rest of my recipes.

One of the greatest things about mineral makeup is its versatility: many of the eye shadows can also be used as eyeliner, and some make great bronzers or highlighters, too. You can even use some eye products on your lips! Just make sure all the micas and pigments you use are approved for safe use on the lips. (For more information on lip-safe ingredients, see page 189.) Because so many mineral makeup products can be used in multiple ways, my recipes include at-a-glance tips for alternative uses.

PRO TIP

TRUE COLORS

The mica and pigment names I use in the following recipes are general and descriptive to help you understand what colors you'll be creating. Many vendors sell similar colors under different names. The Mica and Pigment Substitutions Made Easy chart (page 234) lists some of the names vendors use for these colors, though their actual colors may vary slightly from what I show here. To help you match as closely as possible the micas and pigments I use, refer to the chart on pages 30–31.

In addition, the recipes in this book use small quantities and specify the volume, not weight, of each ingredient. Once you master a technique, you can adjust these recipes to specify weights, which will help you more accurately replicate your results in the future.

TYPES OF MAKEUP DEFINED

BLUSH is a pink, red, and sometimes purple product that gives cheeks a healthy flush of color.

BRONZER is a brown, tan, or bronze makeup product that adds the appearance of depth to the face and/or gives skin a sun-kissed look. To achieve that desirable golden effect, you can use either a shimmery or matte bronzer. You can also use bronzer instead of blush for a more natural golden cheek color. If you want to use bronzer to contour — shading areas of your face to draw attention to certain features and away from others — be sure to use only a matte version.

COLOR CORRECTOR is a pastel-colored product used to counterbalance severe skin discoloration. For example, green color corrector counteracts redness from acne or dryness; yellow counteracts violet under-eye circles, veins, or birthmarks; purple counteracts yellowness and brightens sallow skin; and orange brightens up any bluish discoloration or birthmarks. Color correctors are only needed in extreme cases and should be used underneath concealer and foundation.

CONCEALER is a skin-colored cosmetic designed to cover skin imperfections. Most often concealer is used to mask blemishes or under-eye darkness, but it can also even out eyelid darkness, highlight the face, prime the lips so that lip color adheres better, and mask any discoloration or scarring. If your skin is mostly flawless, you can skip foundation altogether and cover any imperfections with a little concealer and finishing powder.

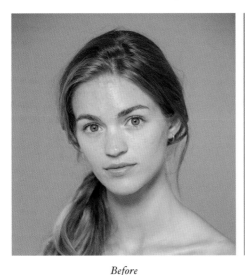

Before

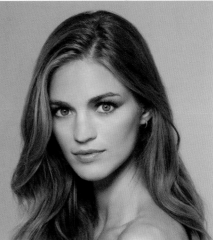

After, with foundation, bronzer, eye shadow, eyeliner, and lip gloss

EYEBROW POWDER is deeply pigmented makeup used to fill in and shape the eyebrows. It is usually a black, brown, or tan color and is always matte. Eyebrow powder can also be used as eyeliner.

EYELINER is a darkly pigmented product used to outline and shape the eyes. It usually comes in black, brown, and blue, but it can be any color you like. Eyeliner can serve as a crease color for a smoky-eye look or as an eyebrow powder if it has a matte finish.

EYE SHADOW is makeup used to color the eyelid. It is usually less pigmented than eyeliner, but eye shadow can be used as an eyeliner when applied wet and with an angled brush.

FINISHING POWDER is a transparent powder that helps makeup last longer. It can be used throughout the day to freshen up makeup and keep oily skin in check.

FOUNDATION is a skin-colored makeup product worn to even out skin texture and color. Usually foundation is used on skin with "imperfections" — such as acne, discoloration, scarring, uneven texture, or freckles — to turn the face into a flawless canvas on which to apply makeup. Foundation can be liquid, cream, tinted moisturizer, or powdered. It offers less color and coverage than concealer or color corrector, so it can be used instead of concealer to even out minor skin flaws or instead of color corrector to balance mild skin discoloration.

HIGHLIGHTER gives the face a glow or dewy complexion and draws attention to wherever it is placed. It is usually a gold, nude, white, or pink color. Highlighter can be worn as an eye shadow or mixed with lip gloss to add a bit of shine as long as the pigments are lip-safe.

LIP BALM is a moisturizing and healing salve that nourishes and conditions the lips. It is usually uncolored and less shiny than lip gloss. Lip balm can be used under lip gloss or alone to moisturize and protect the lips.

LIP GLOSS is a shiny and sticky product that colors and enhances the lips. It can be used alone or with lip balm.

MIXING MEDIUM is a clear solution used to turn powdered cosmetics into cream or liquid makeup. It can also serve as a setting spray or moisturizing spray. When combined with colored powders, mixing medium helps makeup last longer and makes colors brighter and stronger.

PRO TIP

TROUBLESHOOTING COLOR BALANCE

PROBLEM	SOLUTION
Too red	Add green.
Too yellow	Add violet.
Too blue	Add orange.
Too green	Add red.
Too violet	Add yellow.
Too orange	Add blue.
Too light	Add black or more pigments.
Too dark	Add white.
Color too intense	Add sericite.
Color too sheer	Add more pigments.
Color streaks	Blend longer.
Too sparkly	Add more clay or matte sericite.
Too matte	Add mica or lustrous sericite.

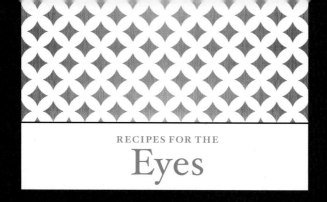

RECIPES FOR THE

Eyes

Each of the eye shadow, eyeliner, eyebrow powder, and highlighter recipes in this section starts with one of two makeup bases. The base you use will depend on whether you want to keep your powders loose or press them into makeup pans. The ratios here will ensure that you get the perfect consistency, no matter how big or small a batch you want to make. To start, I recommend using a teaspoon to measure the parts; this will yield a little less than ¼ cup (60 milliliters) of finished base. Both of the following makeup base recipes should be mixed mechanically.

MAKEUP BASE FOR LOOSE POWDERS

If you plan on leaving your mineral makeup product loose, use this makeup base.

6   parts sericite
2   parts titanium dioxide or zinc oxide
1   part kaolin
1   part magnesium stearate

1. Combine all the ingredients in your mixing container.

2. Blend mechanically for 4 minutes.

MAKEUP BASE FOR PRESSED POWDERS

f you want to press your makeup product, use this recipe for your makeup base.
Some of the following ingredients are available with surface treatments like wax
or the amino acid L-lysine, which will help the powders bind together and press
with ease.

- **6 parts sericite**
- **2 parts zinc oxide**
- **1 part kaolin**
- **1 part magnesium myristate**
- **1 part zinc stearate**

1. Combine all the ingredients in your mixing container.

2. Blend mechanically for 4 minutes.

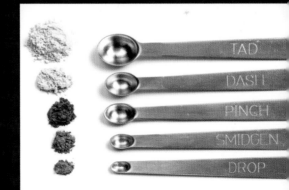

MEASURING KEY	
Tad	¼ teaspoon
Dash	⅛ teaspoon
Pinch	1/16 teaspoon
Smidgen	1/32 teaspoon
Drop	1/64 teaspoon

Note: For best results, use
level spoonfuls.

SHIMMERY EYE SHADOWS

The first mineral makeup I made was sparkly eye shadow. Once I learned how, I was addicted! I started with a few ingredients, and that weekend alone, I created about 60 different eye shadow colors and used up my whole supply of ingredients.

When you are playing around with colors, be sure to save all your creations. Sometimes, if I decide I don't need a color I made, or I choose to tweak the formula, I like to give the originals to friends and family as gifts. I also have a big jar where I pour my "mistakes." Any time I create a color I don't love, instead of throwing it away, I pour it into the big jar with all my other mistakes. Once the jar is full, I mix it well and then press all of the powder into eye shadows. It usually turns out to be a taupe brown shade.

Shimmery eye shadows are relatively easy to prepare, as all you need are a few ingredients that you can mix in a jar, by hand, or in a resealable plastic bag. To make sure your eye shadows have great sparkle, mix the micas in by hand. See pages 202–204 for application tips.

Each of the shimmery eye shadow recipes in the following section makes enough to fill one 5-gram jar.

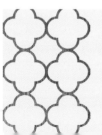

BEAUTY SPOT
EYE SHADOWS SIMPLIFIED

In many eye shadow recipes you find elsewhere, the ratio of makeup base to mica powder is anywhere from 1:1 to 1:3. I personally prefer much more mica than base, as it results

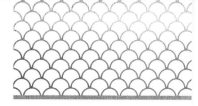

LOOKS GREAT WITH

Skin undertone: Neutral

Eye color: Any

Other uses: Highlighter, lip color

One of the first eye shadows I ever made was a pink-and-blue powder that I called Fairy Floss, since it reminded me of cotton candy or bubble-gum ice cream. I love the name and wanted to create another eye shadow similar to my first.

FAIRY FLOSS

This is a muted pink ivory with a satin-suede finish and silver sparkles. For a casual day look, apply Fairy Floss all over the eyelid.

- 1 dash satin white mica
- 1 pinch plus 1 smidgen satin beige mica
- 1 pinch satin gold mica
- 1 smidgen Makeup Base (page 82 or 83)

Blend together using your preferred mixing method (page 66).

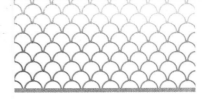

LOOKS GREAT WITH

Skin undertone: Warm and neutral

Eye color: Any, but especially blue or gray

Other uses: Highlighter, blush

BRIAR

This eye shadow is a taupe brown with a gold sparkle. Apply all over the eyelid for a casual day look or wear as a mid-tone color for a smoky-eye look. Briar looks amazing on all skin shades and makes a beautiful highlighter for medium-dark skin shades.

1 pinch plus 1 smidgen silver gold mica
1 pinch nude silver mica
1 pinch satin bronze mica
1 pinch white gold mica
1 smidgen Makeup Base (page 82 or 83)

Blend together using your preferred mixing method (page 66).

I don't usually read fiction, but when I do, I love classic fairy tales that are made modern. Sleeping Beauty and Briar Rose are among my favorites. I love Briar's kind, loving heart; she is incredibly sweet and makes friends with everyone — even woodland creatures! She is the kind of person who will do anything to help someone and make peace. She is a ladylike, classic beauty.

Zephorah is wearing

EYES: Briar and Peacock shadows; Peacock eyeliner; Brunette eyebrow powder

LIPS: Basic Lip Gloss mixed with salmon mica

FACE: Nutmeg–Cream Puff foundation mixture (50:50); Caramel contour; Coral blush; Heatherbelle highlighter

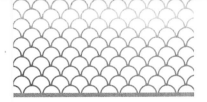

LOOKS GREAT WITH

Skin undertone: Neutral

Eye color: Any

Other uses: Highlighter, bronzer, lip color

BEACH BUNNY

This eye shadow is a creamy pale latte color with a satin finish. It's perfect for a "barely there" eyelid color or as a mid tone for a smoky-eye look. Beach Bunny can be worn as a bronzer for the palest skin colors or as a highlighter for medium-dark skin colors.

   1 pinch plus 1 smidgen muted gold mica

   1 pinch plus 1 smidgen satin bronze mica

   1 pinch satin gold mica

   1 smidgen satin white mica

   1 smidgen Makeup Base (page 82 or 83)

Blend together using your preferred mixing method (page 66).

One of my best friends growing up, Mina, was from Korea. She introduced me to Japanese *manga* comics, where I learned the term *beach bunny* to describe well-tanned girls who hung around the beach. The name is meant as an insult, as women with fair skin are thought to be more beautiful in Japan, but I always found the name cute.

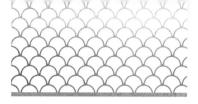

LOOKS GREAT WITH

Skin undertone: Neutral

Eye color: Any

Other uses: Eyeliner,
highlighter, bronzer

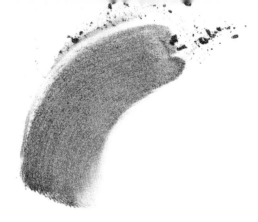

CLANCY

When I was in my first semester of college, I met a boy who changed my life. I had grown up in big cities and my family moved every couple years, but Clancy had lived in the same small town all his life. One day he offered to give me a ride home from school so I wouldn't have to ride the public bus. There was a mix-up with room numbers and since I didn't have a cell phone at the time, I ended up just going home. Later I learned that he had waited for me at school for three hours. It was then I realized he was a keeper. He was my first love and is my soul mate.

This eye shadow is a medium satin milk-chocolate brown with a silver luster. It can be worn as an allover eyelid color for a day look or as a mid-tone shade for a brown smoky-eye look. This color can also serve as a highlighter on very dark skin.

- 1 pinch metallic olive mica
- 1 pinch nude silver mica
- 1 pinch satin bronze mica
- 1 pinch smoky blue mica
- 1 pinch smoky gold mica
- 1 smidgen Makeup Base (page 82 or 83)

Blend together using your preferred mixing method (page 66).

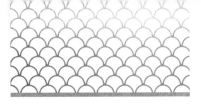

LOOKS GREAT WITH
Skin undertone: Warm
Eye color: Any, but best with
    blue
Other uses: Eyeliner, high-
    lighter, blush, bronzer

CREAM SODA

For a sun-kissed look, wear this eye shadow all over the lid. It also makes a perfect bronzer for pale skin colors and works great as a highlighter for dark skin.

- 1 dash plus 1 smidgen satin bronze mica
- 1 pinch satin gold mica
- 1 smidgen metallic gold mica
- 1 smidgen smoky gold mica
- 1 smidgen Makeup Base (page 82 or 83)

Blend together using your preferred mixing method (page 66).

When I was a kid, my family would go on bike rides to delis and soda shops. There was one in particular where I remember getting root beer floats and cream sodas. This satiny foxtail-bronze eye shadow reminds me of my childhood treats.

Lucy is wearing

EYES: Cream Soda and Calgary shadows; Calgary eyeliner; Oak eyebrow powder

LIPS: Basic Lip Gloss mixed with salmon mica

FACE: Cake foundation; Honey bronzer; Coral blush; Bombshell highlighter

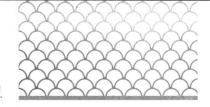

UNDINE

This satiny gray-taupe eye shadow has silver sparkles and is perfect mixed with a darker gray for a smoky-eye look. It also makes a great pale eyeliner for blue or gray eyes.

1 pinch plus 1 smidgen satin gold mica
1 pinch plus 1 smidgen satin white mica
1 pinch smoky blue mica
1 smidgen Makeup Base (page 82 or 83)

Blend together using your preferred mixing method (page 66).

I love sad fairy tales. I don't know why, but tragic romance seems more realistic and relatable to me than "happily ever after." Undine is an old German fairy tale about a water sprite who tragically falls in love with a king. I first heard of Undine in a heartbreaking romance novel called *Haunted Waters*, by Mary Pope Osborne. When I imagine Undine's essence, I see a smoky and mysterious pale grayish green, like the color of this eye shadow.

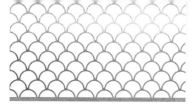

My favorite character in the
King Arthur stories is Morgan
le Fay, even though she is sup-
posed to be the villain. She is
the beautiful star of Nancy
Springer's novel *I Am Morgan
le Fay.* In the book, she tries to
keep the wounded knight she
loves safe in a magical world,
but the knight's need to protect
others eventually pushes her to
set him free and possibly lose
him forever. It's my favorite
part of the book — and it breaks
my heart.

MORGAN LE FAY

This eye shadow is a coppery gold-
amber color. It is pretty when applied
dry but looks even better applied wet.
Mix it with water or a mixing medium
to make the color even more metallic
and intense! Morgan le Fay makes a
hypnotizing and intense eyeliner. To use
it as an eyeliner, mix a bit of the powder
with water or mixing medium until a
cream forms, then apply on your lash
line with an angled brush.

   1 dash metallic gold mica
   1 pinch plus 1 smidgen metallic olive mica
   1 pinch metallic orange mica
   1 smidgen Makeup Base (page 82 or 83)

Blend together using your preferred mixing
method (page 66).

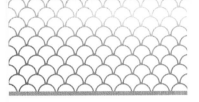

Skin undertone: Cool and
neutral

Eye color: Green, hazel, or
brown

Other uses: Eyeliner

FERN GULLY

Fern Gully is a golden olive powder that can be worn as an allover lid color. It also works as a light eyeliner, and you can apply it with a wet brush to darken the color.

1 dash satin gold mica
1 pinch plus 1 smidgen muted gold mica
1 smidgen satin black mica
1 smidgen smoky green mica
1 smidgen Makeup Base (page 82 or 83)

Blend together using your preferred mixing method (page 66).

I love moss, ferns, and all the other greenery I remember from my childhood in Michigan. Now that I live in Utah, I miss foggy afternoons and the slick, mossy rocks and ferns in our front garden.

Sahira is wearing

EYES: Fern Gully shadow; Fireflies eyeliner; Brunette eyebrow powder

FACE: Caramel foundation; bright red mica blush

LIPS: Ruby Red

STARGIRL

This eye shadow is a satiny smooth bronzed gold with subtle silver specks. For a soft daytime look, use Stargirl dry, applying it either to the outer corners of the eyelids or in the crease of the eyelids. For a bolder metallic eyeshadow or eyeliner, apply wet.

    1 pinch metallic olive mica
    1 pinch metallic orange mica
    1 pinch muted gold mica
    1 pinch pink blue mica
    1 pinch satin gold mica
    1 smidgen Makeup Base (page 82 or 83)

Blend together using your preferred mixing method (page 66).

One of my favorite books is *Stargirl*, by Jerry Spinelli. The title character is described this way: "She was elusive. She was today. She was tomorrow. She was the faintest scent of a cactus flower, the flitting shadow of an elf owl. We did not know what to make of her. In our minds we tried to pin her to a corkboard like a butterfly, but the pin merely went through and away she flew." Stargirl reminds me of the good in the world. Her childlike innocence and happiness brighten the dark gray muddy world.

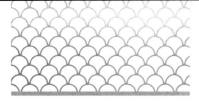

LOOKS GREAT WITH

Skin undertone: Cool
Eye color: Blue, gray, or brown
Other uses: Eyeliner

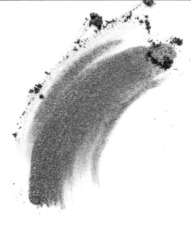

ECHO

In middle school one of my history teachers often used an old tape recorder and slide projector in class to give lessons on Greek mythology. My favorite myth was about the nymph named Echo and her unwavering love for a handsome young man named Narcissus.

This eye shadow is a sparkly, smoky steel gray with inky blue hints. It's best for nighttime wear, and makes a beautiful smoky-eye look when used as the mid-tone or darkest shade. It also creates a fun twist on the cat-eye winged look. For an intense lustrous eyeliner, apply Echo wet using a slanted brush.

> 1 pinch plus 1 smidgen smoky blue mica
> 1 pinch glimmering white mica
> 1 pinch satin black mica
> 1 pinch muted silver mica
> 1 smidgen Makeup Base (page 82 or 83)

Blend together using your preferred mixing method (page 66).

MATTE EYE SHADOWS

Matte eye shadow is currently in style, as it looks somewhat more natural than shimmery eye shadow. It's perfect for easygoing day looks and can be worn alone, with other matte shadows, or mixed with lustrous eye shadows for more dimension.

These recipes include a small amount of sericite to fluff up the powders, as matte pigments on their own tend to be dense, intense, and hard to spread. If your shadows are too saturated, you can always add some sericite to lighten them and add sheerness. Always remember to grind the matte shadows in a mechanical grinder. See pages 202–204 for application tips.

Each of the matte eye shadow recipes in the following section makes enough to fill one 5-gram jar.

BEAUTY SPOT

UNIVERSALLY FLATTERING EYE SHADOWS

No matter what color skin, hair, or eyes you have, you'll look great in:

- Fairy Floss (page 85)
- Cream Soda (page 90)
- Undine (page 92)
- Echo (page 97)
- Buttercream (page 99)
- Bones (page 106)
- Rueger (page 108)
- Calgary (page 110)

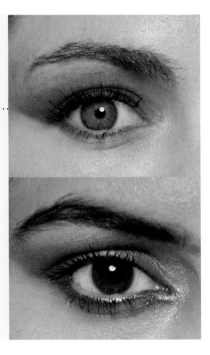

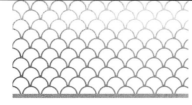

Skin undertone: Warm

Eye color: Any

Other uses: Highlighter, foundation

BUTTERCREAM

This is a creamy nude ivory that works great as a pale eyelid color for daytime looks or paired with a classic black winged eyeliner. It's perfect for a matte under-brow arch color or to lighten around the corner of the eyes.

- 1 tad Makeup Base (page 82 or 83)
- 1 tad sericite
- 1 pinch titanium dioxide
- 1 smidgen ultramarine pink
- 1 smidgen yellow iron oxide

1. Combine the Makeup Base and sericite in your mixing container.

2. Blend mechanically for 30 seconds, then add the remaining ingredients on the list, blending for 30 seconds after each addition.

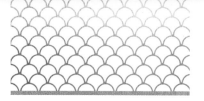

LOOKS GREAT WITH
Skin undertone: Warm and
  neutral
Eye color: Blue or brown
Other uses: Eyebrow powder,
  foundation, bronzer

BAMBI

This creamy and pale terra-cotta–pink eye shadow works best
with blue eyes. It can be worn as an allover eyelid color or just
in the crease for a warm flash of color.

1 tad Makeup Base (page 82
  or 83)

1 tad sericite

1 dash yellow iron oxide

1 pinch titanium dioxide

1 smidgen manganese violet

1 drop red iron oxide

1 drop ultramarine blue

1. Combine the Makeup Base and sericite
    in your mixing container.

2. Blend mechanically for 30 seconds,
    then add the remaining ingredients on
    the list, blending for 30 seconds after
    each addition.

Carly is wearing

EYES: Bambi and Briar shadows

LIPS: Basic Lip Gloss mixed with salmon mica and Wonderland

FACE: Cake and Honey foundation; Coral blush; Heatherbelle highlighter

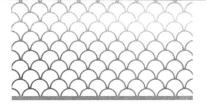

LOOKS GREAT WITH
Skin undertone: Warm
Eye color: Any
Other uses: Eyeliner, eyebrow
    powder, foundation, blush,
    bronzer

RED VELVET

As a matte cinnamon brown, this works best for evening looks and makes a perfect mid-tone color for a smoky-eye look. You can apply it to the corner or crease of the eyelid for a vamp look. Red Velvet can be used as an eyeliner or, for medium-dark skin colors, as a bronzer or blush.

1 tad Makeup Base (page 82
    or 83)
1 tad sericite
1 pinch hydrated chromium oxide
    green
1 smidgen manganese violet
1 smidgen red iron oxide
1 smidgen yellow iron oxide

1. Combine the Makeup Base and sericite in your mixing container.

2. Blend mechanically for 30 seconds, then add the remaining ingredients on the list, blending for 30 seconds after each addition.

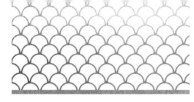

LOOKS GREAT WITH

Skin undertone: Cool and
  neutral

Eye color: Any

Other uses: Eyeliner, eyebrow
  powder, foundation, bronzer

OAK

Best worn for an evening look, this medium brown eye shadow has a warm undertone. It can be applied as an allover eyelid color, in the outer corner of the eyelids, or as a mid-tone color for a smoky-eye look. Oak can also be worn as a soft eyeliner color or as a bronzer for medium-dark skin shades.

1 pinch Makeup Base (page 82 or 83)

1 pinch sericite

1 pinch chromium oxide green

1 smidgen red iron oxide

1 smidgen titanium dioxide

1 smidgen ultramarine blue

1 smidgen yellow iron oxide

1. Combine the Makeup Base and sericite in your mixing container.

2. Blend mechanically for 30 seconds, then add the remaining ingredients on the list, blending for 30 seconds after each addition.

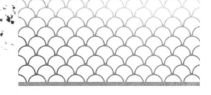

LOOKS GREAT WITH

Skin undertone: Cool and
neutral

Eye color: Any

Other uses: Eyeliner, eyebrow
powder, foundation,
bronzer

BONSAI

This soft charcoal-brown color is perfect
for evening looks. It can be used as a
crease color when doing a smoky-eye
look or as a soft-smudged eyeliner
applied with a dry brush. When applied
with a wet brush, Bonsai also works well
as a black-brown eyeliner.

Bonsai trees are perfect. I have
always loved miniature things,
and I think bonsai gardens and
glass terrariums are some of the
most magical creations ever.

1 tad Makeup Base (page 82 or 83)

1 tad sericite

1 pinch black iron oxide

1 smidgen chromium oxide green

1 smidgen red iron oxide

1 smidgen ultramarine blue

1 smidgen yellow iron oxide

1. Combine the Makeup Base and sericite in your
    mixing container.

2. Blend mechanically for 30 seconds, then add
    the remaining ingredients on the list, blending
    for 30 seconds after each addition.

Germaine is wearing

EYES: Buttercream, Oak, and Bonsai shadows; Bonsai eyeliner

LIPS: Basic Lip Gloss mixed with salmon mica

FACE: Eggnog foundation; Suede bronzer

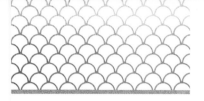

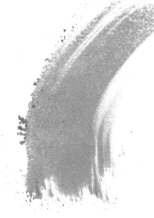

LOOKS GREAT WITH

Skin undertone: Cool and
  neutral
Eye color: Any, but especially
  blue or gray
Other uses: Eyebrow powder

BONES

This soft ashy taupe is gorgeous as an
allover lid color for day and night looks.

  1 tad Makeup Base (page 82 or 83)
  1 tad sericite
  1 dash ultramarine pink
  1 pinch titanium dioxide
  1 pinch yellow iron oxide
  1 smidgen black iron oxide

1. Combine the Makeup Base and sericite in your
    mixing container.

2. Blend mechanically for 30 seconds, then add
    the remaining ingredients on the list, blending
    for 30 seconds after each addition.

The first concert I ever
attended was by the Killers, a
Las Vegas–based rock band. I
wish I had the talent to write
beautiful, relatable, and poetic
verses like the Killers do. I
especially love their songs
"Bones," "Smile Like You Mean
It," and "A Dustland Fairytale."
Nothing is better than a song
with good lyrics.

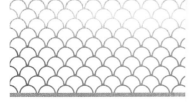

LOOKS GREAT WITH

Skin undertone: Cool

Eye color: Green or hazel

Other uses: Eyeliner

CASHMERE

This dusty and muted mauve eye shadow looks best as an allover eyelid color.

I love clothing but am a frugal person, so I often hunt for treasures at thrift stores. The first cashmere item I ever bought was a secondhand sweater. When I found it, I instantly fell in love with how soft and luxurious it felt. I now have one other cashmere sweater, but I can't wait for the day when I can afford a collection of cashmere scarves and sweaters. That will be a happy day.

1 pinch Makeup Base (page 82 or 83)

1 pinch sericite

1 pinch plus 1 smidgen manganese violet

1 pinch titanium dioxide

1 pinch ultramarine pink

1 smidgen hydrated chromium oxide green

1 smidgen yellow iron oxide

1. Combine the Makeup Base and sericite in your mixing container.

2. Blend mechanically for 30 seconds, then add the remaining ingredients on the list, blending for 30 seconds after each addition.

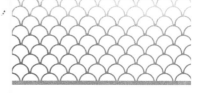

LOOKS GREAT WITH

Skin undertone: Cool
Eye color: Blue or brown
Other uses: Eyeliner, eyebrow
    powder

RUEGER

This eye shadow is a smoky dark steel gray with hints of blue. Use it as a crease color for a black or silver smoky-eye look. It also makes a perfect dark gray eyeliner, and you can apply it dry or wet.

If I ever have a boy, I would love to call him Rueger. It's just a good name.

1 tad Makeup Base (page 82 or 83)
1 tad sericite
1 dash plus 1 smidgen black iron oxide
1 pinch plus 1 smidgen yellow iron oxide
1 pinch ultramarine blue

1. Combine the Makeup Base and sericite in your mixing container.

2. Blend mechanically for 30 seconds, then add the remaining ingredients on the list, blending for 30 seconds after each addition.

Lakshmi is wearing

EYES: Echo, Rueger, and Undine shadows; Echo eyeliner; Fireflies eyebrow powder

LIPS: Girl Crush

FACE: Honey foundation; Coral blush; Flurries highlighter

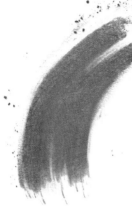

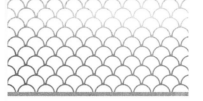

CALGARY

Somewhere between mauve, taupe, and brown, this eye shadow is best for evening looks. It is beautiful as an allover eyelid color.

- 1 pinch Makeup Base (page 82 or 83)
- 1 pinch sericite
- 1 pinch plus 1 smidgen manganese violet
- 1 pinch chromium oxide green
- 1 smidgen red iron oxide

1. Combine the Makeup Base and sericite in your mixing container.

2. Blend mechanically for 30 seconds, then add the remaining ingredients on the list, blending for 30 seconds after each addition.

For two years, I wished I were in Calgary, Alberta. My boyfriend had gone to Canada for a religious mission, and he wasn't allowed to make phone calls, Skype, or have regular contact with anyone at home. So we wrote letters. I sent hundreds of decorated, stickered, glittery, brightly colored letters. Sometimes they included mini-cassette recordings of me just talking about life and telling him stories. Communication has evolved so much in the past few years, and I sometimes miss the old-fashioned letter.

SHIMMERY EYELINERS

I love shimmery eyeliners, as they make any day or night a little more glamorous. Although you can use any shimmery eye shadow as an eyeliner, these recipes are formulated to offer the most pigmentation and sparkle. They can be applied either dry or wet. If you want a long-lasting nighttime look, you can use these eyeliners wet as an allover eyelid color. See pages 204–205 for application tips.

Each of the shimmery eyeliner recipes in the following section makes enough to fill one 10-gram jar.

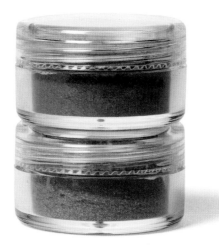

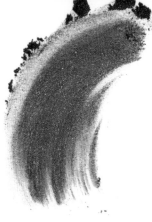

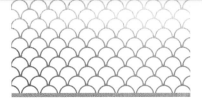

LOOKS GREAT WITH
Skin undertone: Warm
Eye color: Any, but especially
  green
Other uses: Eye shadow, lip
  color, bronzer

KITTY-CAT

This plum-brown eyeliner has aqua sparkles. It can be applied wet or dry and makes an interesting winged eyeliner look.

1 dash Makeup Base (page 82 or 83)

1 smidgen black iron oxide

1 smidgen red iron oxide

1 tad glimmering brown blue mica

1 tad satin brown blue mica

1. Combine the Makeup Base and black iron oxide in your mixing container.

2. Blend mechanically for 30 seconds, then add the red iron oxide and blend for an additional 30 seconds.

3. Incorporate the micas by hand with your mixing method of choice (page 66).

Veronica is wearing

EYES: Calgary, Red Velvet, Wonderland, and Fairy Floss shadows; Kitty-Cat eyeliner

LIPS: Basic Lip Gloss mixed with Vamp

FACE: Cream Puff foundation; Suede bronzer; Cherry Blossom blush; Wonderland highlighter

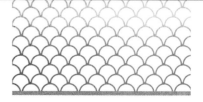

LOOKS GREAT WITH
Skin undertone: Neutral
Eye color: Any
Other uses: Eye shadow,
bronzer, lip color

SEQUINS

This champagne-brown eyeliner with silver sparkles looks amazing applied wet, which makes it appear even more metallic. It makes a perfect foiled eye shadow when applied wet. You can also apply it dry as an eyeliner or eye shadow.

1 dash Makeup Base (page 82 or 83)

1 smidgen black iron oxide

1 smidgen red iron oxide

1 smidgen yellow iron oxide

1 tad satin bronze mica

1 dash glimmering white mica

1 dash satin gold mica

1 dash silver gold mica

1 dash smoky gold mica

1. Combine the Makeup Base and black iron oxide in your mixing container.

2. Blend mechanically for 30 seconds, then add each iron oxide on the list, blending for 30 seconds after each addition.

3. Incorporate the micas by hand with your mixing method of choice (page 66).

MATTE EYELINERS

Like all mineral powder, this eyeliner powder can be used dry or wet. If you want to add a bit of luster to any of the recipes, first grind the pigments with a mechanical grinder, then gently stir in mica by hand. See pages 204–205 for application tips.

Each of the matte eyeliner recipes in the following section makes enough to fill one 10-gram jar.

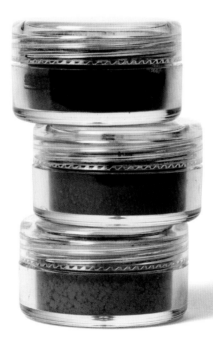

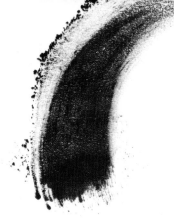

LOOKS GREAT WITH
Skin undertone: Neutral
Eye color: Any
Other uses: Eye shadow,
   eyebrow powder

FIREFLIES

This eyeliner is a deep grayish black that looks great applied dry for a smoky, smudged appearance. You can apply it wet for a dramatic winged look. Fireflies also works well as a smoky-eye shadow color.

I grew up chasing fireflies. Now I live in Utah, where there aren't any. I have to explain to my husband and girls what fireflies are, as if they were mythical creatures the world can only vaguely remember.

½ teaspoon black iron oxide
1 tad Makeup Base (page 82 or 83)
1 pinch red iron oxide
1 pinch ultramarine blue
1 pinch yellow iron oxide

1. Combine the black iron oxide and Makeup Base in your mixing container.

2. Blend mechanically for 30 seconds, then add the remaining ingredients on the list, blending for an additional 30 seconds after each addition.

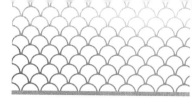

LOOKS GREAT WITH

Skin undertone: Warm

Eye color: Any

Other uses: Eye shadow,
   eyebrow powder

I miss having a real fireplace
and chimney, like we did when
I was a kid. We would gather
wood, start a fire, and warm
the whole house.

CHIMNEY

This deep and warm eyeliner has hints
of purple with a mixture of red, black,
and brown that reminds me of the colors
of our old chimney. It looks gorgeous for
any nighttime look and makes a great
smoky eyeliner.

½ teaspoon black iron oxide
  1 tad Makeup Base (page 82 or 83)
  1 dash red iron oxide
  1 dash ultramarine blue
  1 pinch yellow iron oxide

1. Combine the black iron oxide and Makeup
    Base in your mixing container.

2. Blend mechanically for 30 seconds, then add
    the remaining ingredients on the list, blending
    for 30 seconds after each addition.

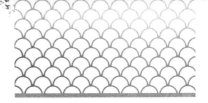

LOOKS GREAT WITH
Skin undertone: Cool
Eye color: Any
Other uses: Eye shadow,
   eyebrow powder

PEACOCK

This true navy-blue eyeliner also makes a dramatic and smoky eye shadow color. It's best for nighttime looks, with a nude lip.

1 tad Makeup Base (page 82 or 83)

1 tad sericite

1 dash black iron oxide

1 dash hydrated chromium oxide green

1 dash ultramarine blue

1. Combine the Makeup Base and sericite in your mixing container.

2. Blend mechanically for 30 seconds, then add the remaining ingredients on the list, blending for 30 seconds after each addition.

Coco is wearing

EYES: Briar and Fern Gully shadows; Peacock eyeliner; Raven eyebrow powder

LIPS: Basic Lip Gloss mixed with Vamp

FACE: Cake foundation; Toffee bronzer; Vamp blush

MATTE EYEBROW POWDERS

Brow powder tends to look more natural than eyebrow pencils, as the powder can fill in sparse eyebrows and subtly darken their color. It tends to exist only in a matte finish, since shimmery eyebrows are not very flattering.

Structured, manicured, bold eyebrows are in high demand these days. With the recipes that follow, you can mix and match colors to get your perfect brow shade. Always apply eyebrow powder with a dry angled eyebrow or eyeliner brush.

Each of the matte eyebrow powder recipes in the following section makes enough to fill one 10-gram jar.

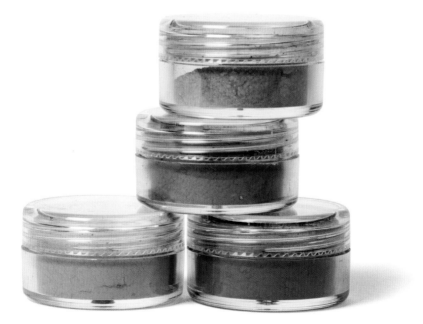

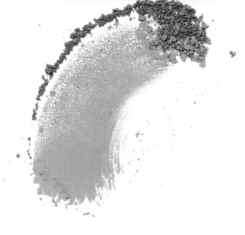

LOOKS GREAT WITH

Skin undertone: Neutral

Other uses: Eye shadow,
   eyeliner, foundation,
   bronzer

BLONDIE

This light golden-brown eyebrow powder can also be used as a
medium brown eyelid color or a bronzer for medium skin colors.

½ teaspoon sericite

1 tad plus 1 smidgen yellow iron
   oxide

1 tad Makeup Base (page 82
   or 83)

1 tad titanium dioxide

1 pinch black iron oxide

1 pinch red iron oxide

1. Combine the sericite and yellow iron
   oxide in your mixing container.

2. Blend mechanically for 30 seconds, then
   add the remaining ingredients on the
   list, blending for 30 seconds after each
   addition.

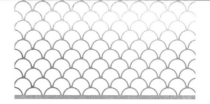

LOOKS GREAT WITH
Skin undertone: Warm
Other uses: Eye shadow,
eyeliner, blush, bronzer

GINGER

The perfect eyebrow color for a strawberry blonde, this can also be used as a dark eye shadow or as a blush for dark skin colors.

½ teaspoon sericite
1 tad Makeup Base (page 82 or 83)
1 dash plus 1 pinch titanium oxide
1 dash yellow iron oxide
1 pinch chromium oxide green
1 pinch red iron oxide

1. Combine the sericite and Makeup Base in your mixing container.

2. Blend mechanically for 30 seconds, then add the remaining ingredients on the list, blending for 30 seconds after each addition.

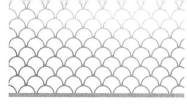

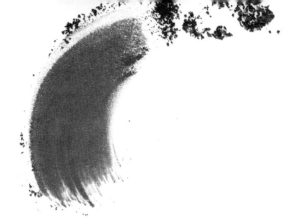

LOOKS GREAT WITH

Skin undertone: Neutral

Other uses: Eye shadow, eyeliner, foundation, bronzer

BRUNETTE

This smoky-brown eyebrow powder can also be worn as a deep brown eyeliner or as the mid-tone or darkest shade when creating a smoky-eye look.

½ teaspoon sericite

1 tad Makeup Base (page 82 or 83)

1 dash yellow iron oxide

1 pinch black iron oxide

1 pinch chromium oxide green

1 pinch red iron oxide

1 pinch ultramarine blue

1. Combine the sericite and Makeup Base in your mixing container.

2. Blend mechanically for 30 seconds, then add the remaining ingredients on the list, blending for 30 seconds after each addition.

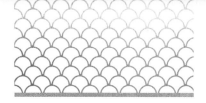

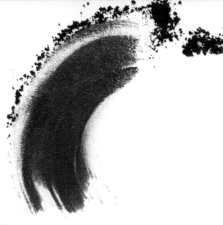

RECIPES FOR THE EYES

LOOKS GREAT WITH

Skin undertone: Neutral

Other uses: Eye shadow,
eyeliner

RAVEN

This black-brown eyebrow powder can be used as a dark eyeliner.
You can also apply it as the darkest eye shadow shade to create a
smoky look.

½ teaspoon sericite

1 tad Makeup Base (page 82
or 83)

1 dash plus 1 pinch black iron
oxide

1 pinch red iron oxide

1 pinch ultramarine blue

1 pinch yellow iron oxide

1. Combine the sericite and Makeup Base
in your mixing container.

2. Blend mechanically for 30 seconds,
then add the remaining ingredients on
the list, blending for 30 seconds after
each addition.

Zephorah is wearing

EYES: Echo shadow;
Raven eyeliner;
Brunette and Raven
eyebrow powders

LIPS: Ruby Red

FACE: Nutmeg–
Cream Puff
foundation mixture
(50:50); Caramel
contour; Coral
blush; Heatherbelle
highlighter

HIGHLIGHTERS

As the name suggests, highlighters attract light and give your face a bright, natural glow. If you are a fan of dewy makeup, you will love using highlighter. You can play around with different mica colors and finishes. For a subtle glow, use finer micas, and for a noticeable sparkle, try larger-particle micas. For pale skin, try white, cream, shimmery gold, or baby pink. For medium and dark skin, try bronze, copper, deep gold, or light tan. See page 208 for application tips.

Each of the highlighter recipes in the following section makes enough to fill one 30-gram jar.

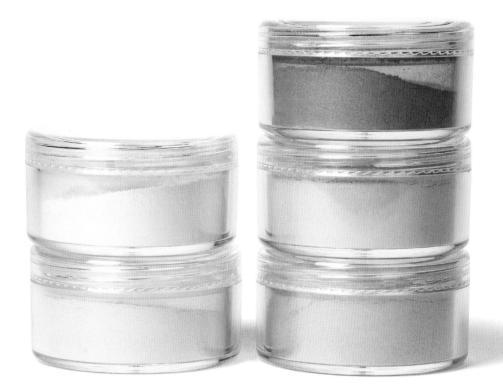

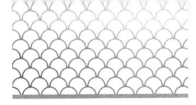

LOOKS GREAT WITH

Skin undertone: Cool and
 neutral

Other uses: Eye shadow

There is something perfect
about flurries in a snow globe:
all the beauty of snow without
all the cold!

FLURRIES

This silvery-white luster can also be used
as a white eye shadow.

 4 teaspoons plus 1 tad satin white mica
 1 tad glimmering white mica
 1 dash Makeup Base (page 82 or 83)

Blend together using your preferred mixing
method (page 66).

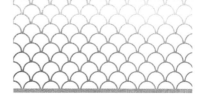

LOOKS GREAT WITH
Skin undertone: Warm
Other uses: Eye shadow

BOMBSHELL

This buttery-gold highlighter can also be worn as a gold eye shadow.

4   teaspoons plus 1 tad white gold mica
1   tad satin gold mica
1   dash Makeup Base (page 82 or 83)

Blend together using your preferred mixing method (page 66).

In school whenever we were assigned to read a biography about a famous person, I always chose Marilyn Monroe. Something about her has always fascinated me. She was glamorous and perfect, unreal in a way, almost not human. She was the closest thing this earth has ever had to a real unicorn.

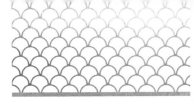

Skin undertone: Cool

Other uses: Eye shadow, lip
    color, blush

I like the idea of an extravagant
and magical otherworld existing
just through a rabbit hole.

WONDERLAND

This blush-pink highlighter has a baby-
blue iridescence. It can also be worn as
a lip gloss or as a two-toned eye shadow.
No matter how you wear it, Wonderland
looks amazing when applied wet!

4½ teaspoons pink-blue mica
    1 dash Makeup Base (page 82 or 83)

Blend together using your preferred mixing
method (page 66).

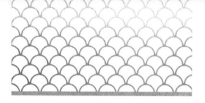

LOOKS GREAT WITH

Skin undertone: Warm

Other uses: Eye shadow

NECTAR

This highlighter is a pastel yellow with a green iridescence, and it can also be worn as a yellow-green eye shadow. It makes an especially gorgeous eye shadow when applied wet.

4½ teaspoons pale yellow-green mica

   1 dash Makeup Base (page 82 or 83)

Blend together using your preferred mixing method (page 66).

This color is what I imagine plants' sugary liquid looks like: warm, radiant, and candylike.

Susannah is wearing

EYES: Fern Gully, Undine, and Nectar shadows; Chimney eyeliner; Blondie eyebrow powder

FACE: Vanilla foundation; Sun-Kissed bronzer; Cupcake blush; Nectar highlighter

LIPS: Foxy

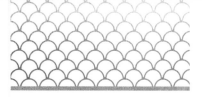

LOOKS GREAT WITH
Skin undertone: Warm
Other uses: Eye shadow, blush,
   lip color

HEATHERBELLE

This peachy highlighter has a golden luster and can be used as a lip gloss or worn as an eye shadow that's perfect for blue eyes!

   1 teaspoon plus 3 dashes peach gold mica
   1 tad plus 1 dash white gold mica
   1 tad satin gold mica
   1 dash Makeup Base (page 82 or 83)

Blend together using your preferred mixing method (page 66).

Most of my family is from the South, and as a kid I was often called Heather Belle. I used to hate the nickname, but now I think it makes my name sound prettier, as *Heather* can be a bit boring. I love so many things about the South, including wraparound porches, fireflies, and the beaches.

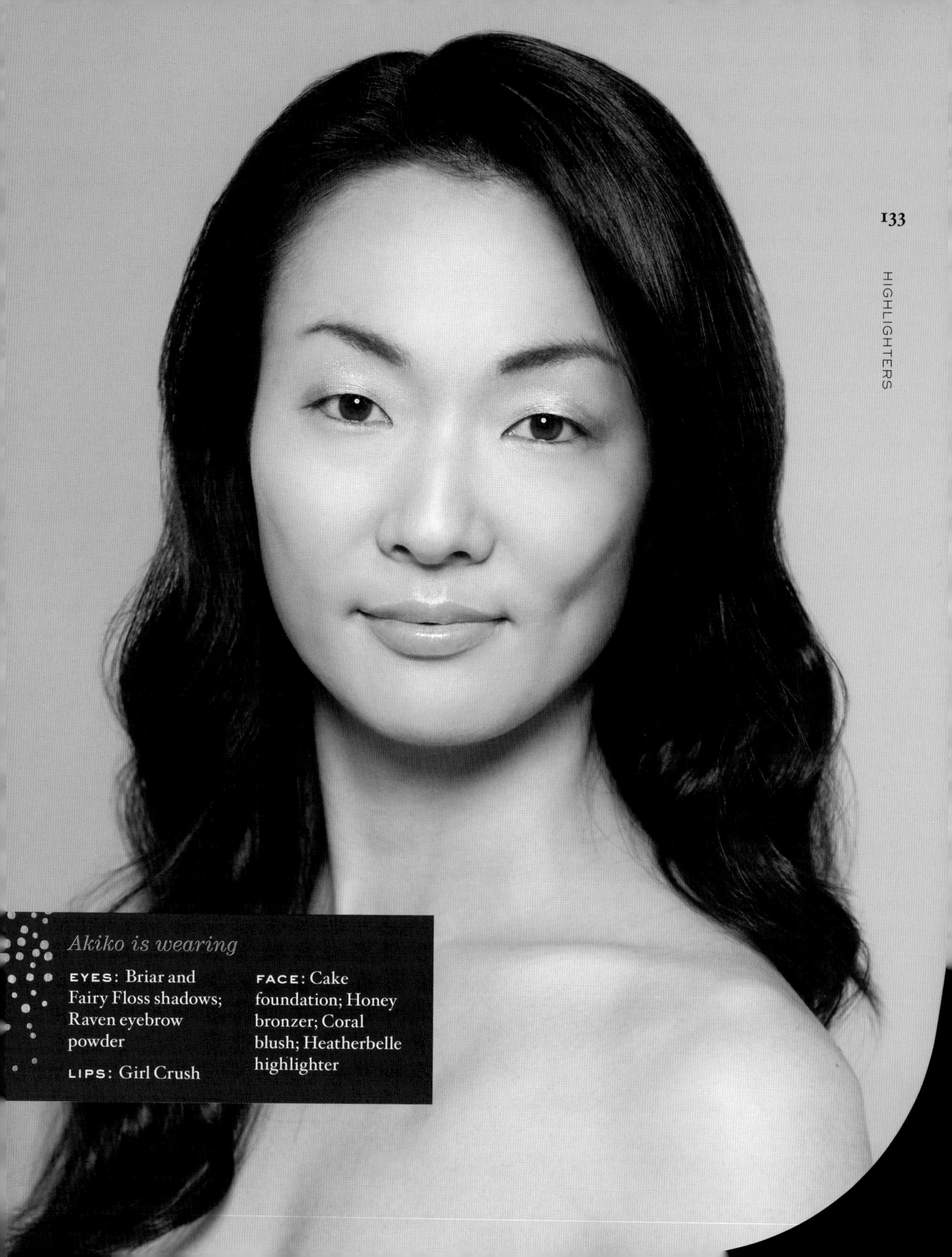

Akiko is wearing

EYES: Briar and
Fairy Floss shadows;
Raven eyebrow
powder

LIPS: Girl Crush

FACE: Cake
foundation; Honey
bronzer; Coral
blush; Heatherbelle
highlighter

Face

After mastering eye makeup, you're ready for the challenge of creating great face cosmetics. Each of the eight foundation base recipes that follows offers unique benefits. Choose the one most appropriate for your skin type.

The most difficult part of making foundation is matching your skin undertone. Once you figure out the right match, you will have a starting place for all your recipes, and when your skin shade changes through the seasons and over the years, you will know how to tweak your formulas.

To start, I suggest making small batches of all of the foundation recipes in your skin shade range and then testing them on your jawline. You might not find an exact match, but choose the closest color.

You can then alter that recipe to match your exact skin shade. If your skin is very light, use fewer pigments and more titanium dioxide. For darker skin, use less titanium dioxide and more pigments. To best match a very dark skin shade, use zinc oxide and/or a combination of yellow, red, and black iron oxide.

In addition to matching your skin color, you should consider your skin's undertone and type. See chapter 2 for more information on undertone, and chapter 3 for details on skin type.

FOUNDATION BASES

I have been making my own foundation for years now and can never go back to traditional store-bought versions. Out of all the cosmetic products I make, formulating my own foundation saves me the most money. And because I put foundation all over my face, it's also the product that offers the biggest benefit to my skin. Many store-bought foundations are full of harsh chemicals and irritants. By making my own, I'm in control of which ingredients I avoid and which I add to soothe my skin.

Each of the foundation base recipes in the following section makes enough to fill one 30-gram jar.

SIMPLE LIGHT FOUNDATION BASE

With only two ingredients, this recipe is perfect for anyone just starting to make cosmetics or for someone seeking a quick and inexpensive alternative to the other makeup bases I include below. As is, this recipe works best for light to medium skin colors.

1 **teaspoon plus 1 tad sericite**

1 **teaspoon plus 1 tad titanium dioxide**

1. Combine the ingredients in your mixing container.

2. Blend mechanically for 4 minutes.

SIMPLE DARK FOUNDATION BASE

The bright mustard-yellow iron oxide in this recipe is perfect for creating makeup for medium to dark skin colors. For more details on how to customize foundation base colors for dark skin, see the sidebar on the facing page.

1½ teaspoons sericite

½ teaspoon yellow iron oxide

½ teaspoon zinc oxide

1. Combine all the ingredients in your mixing container.

2. Blend mechanically for 4 minutes.

NORMAL SKIN FOUNDATION BASE

This foundation base is perfect for those with balanced skin types, as the kaolin offers a small amount of oil control, while the zinc stearate is great for dry skin and acne. As is, it's best for pale to medium-colored skin.

1 teaspoon plus 1 tad sericite

1 teaspoon plus 1 tad titanium dioxide

1 pinch kaolin

1 pinch zinc stearate

1. Combine all the ingredients in your mixing container.

2. Blend mechanically for 4 minutes.

BEAUTY SPOT

DARK FOUNDATION BASE

To create a foundation that matches dark skin, first choose one of the foundation base recipes to best accommodate your skin type. The main thing you will change is the amount of titanium dioxide and zinc oxide. Titanium dioxide is what gives many dark foundations an ashy appearance. If you have medium to dark skin, start by substituting zinc oxide for any titanium dioxide. To darken the foundation from there, substitute yellow iron oxide for half of the zinc oxide. If you find the foundation is still too light or ashy, omit all of the zinc oxide and replace it with yellow iron oxide. For very deep skin colors, add red iron oxide and/or black iron oxide.

You will likely have to experiment with the exact substitution quantities, but one of the benefits of creating your own makeup is that you can match your skin color perfectly. Just be sure to keep track of your ratios until you get a foundation color you're happy with so you can replicate it in the future!

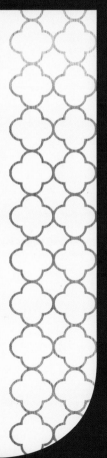

SENSITIVE SKIN FOUNDATION BASE

My skin is very sensitive, and this is the foundation base I use. The allantoin, rice powder, and zinc oxide help in so many ways, protecting the skin from elements and irritants; moisturizing, soothing, and healing the skin; and encouraging cell turnover and skin growth. If your skin isn't sensitive all the time, use this foundation base while you're healing from any kind of skin injury, including chemical peels, microdermabrasion, or facial surgery.

1   teaspoon plus 1 tad zinc oxide
1   teaspoon sericite
1   dash rice powder
1   smidgen cornstarch
1   drop allantoin
1   drop calcium carbonate
1   drop zinc stearate

1. Combine all the ingredients in your mixing container.

2. Blend mechanically for 4 minutes.

MATURE SKIN FOUNDATION BASE

Some people don't consider mature skin to be an actual skin type, but I created this foundation to help minimize fine lines.

1   teaspoon plus 1 tad sericite
1   teaspoon titanium dioxide
1   pinch silica
1   smidgen magnesium stearate
1   drop magnesium myristate
1   dash satin white mica

1. Combine all the ingredients except the silica and mica in your mixing container.

2. Blend mechanically for 4 minutes.

3. Incorporate the silica and mica by hand with your preferred mixing method (page 66).

OILY SKIN FOUNDATION BASE

Powdered mineral makeup generally works really well on oily skin, but when you add some absorbing ingredients like kaolin and arrowroot powder, you get flawless, shine-free skin. The zinc oxide in this recipe helps soothe and heal acne.

½ teaspoon plus 1 tad sericite

½ teaspoon plus 1 tad titanium dioxide

½ teaspoon arrowroot powder

1 tad rice powder

1 drop calcium carbonate

1 drop kaolin

1 drop silica

1. Combine all the ingredients except the silica in your mixing container.

2. Blend mechanically for 4 minutes.

3. Incorporate the silica by hand with your preferred mixing method (page 66).

DRY SKIN FOUNDATION BASE

The L-lysine–treated sericite in this recipe helps prevent moisture from leaving the skin. To further combat dry skin, you can mix this foundation with a glycerin-based setting spray or water and then apply, or lightly mist your face once you have finished applying the powder.

1 **teaspoon L-lysine–treated sericite**

1 **teaspoon titanium dioxide**

1 **tad allantoin**

1 **tad zinc stearate**

1 **drop magnesium myristate**

1 **drop magnesium stearate**

1. Combine all the ingredients in your mixing container.

2. Blend mechanically for 4 minutes.

DEWY SKIN FOUNDATION BASE

This foundation base is great for those with flawless skin. The mica gives it a velvety finish with just a hint of radiance and shimmer, while the silica smooths out the appearance of fine lines. When my skin is doing its best, I like to draw attention to it with this satiny foundation base.

1 **teaspoon titanium dioxide**

1 **teaspoon zinc oxide**

1 **tad L-lysine–treated sericite**

1 **dash magnesium myristate**

1 **dash silica-treated sericite**

1 **pinch zinc stearate**

1 **dash satin white mica**

1. Combine all the ingredients except the silica-treated sericite and mica in your mixing container.

2. Blend mechanically for 4 minutes.

3. Incorporate the silica-treated sericite and mica by hand with your preferred mixing method (page 66).

FOUNDATIONS

One of the biggest complaints I hear about store-bought foundation is the poor color selection. Unless you have medium-light or medium skin, your options are very limited. When I used to buy foundation, I could only ever find one color that was light enough for my pale skin, and even that was way too pink for my warm undertones. I know many women of color who can find only one or two foundations that are even close to their skin tones, but often even those result in an unpleasant ashy look.

When you make your own makeup, you have the power to match your skin shade and undertones perfectly. Although it does take some practice, with time you will be able to find a fantastic match, and there is nothing more rewarding! Use the recipes that follow as a starting place. From there you can combine foundation colors or alter formulas as needed to match your skin. See pages 205–206 for application tips.

Each of the foundation recipes in the following section makes enough to fill one 30-gram jar.

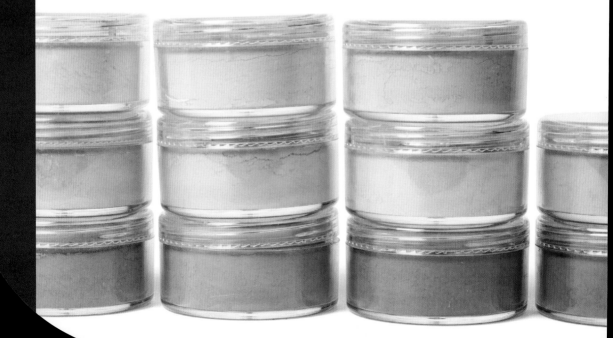

LOOKS GREAT WITH

Skin undertone: Warm and
   neutral
Other uses: Eye shadow

VANILLA

With hints of peaches and cream, this foundation also works well as
a pale matte eye shadow.

2½ teaspoons any white foundation
   base (pages 135–141)
1 tad titanium dioxide
1 dash plus 1 smidgen yellow iron
   oxide
1 drop red iron oxide
1 drop ultramarine blue

1. Combine the foundation base and titanium dioxide in your mixing container.

2. Blend mechanically for 1 minute.

3. Add the remaining ingredients on
   the list, blending for 1 minute after
   each addition.

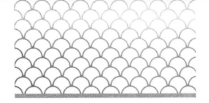

LOOKS GREAT WITH
Skin undertone: Warm
Other uses: Eye shadow

EGGNOG

This golden-ginger foundation can double as a pale matte beige eye shadow.

2½ teaspoons any white foundation base (pages 135–141)
1 tad yellow iron oxide
1 dash titanium dioxide
1 drop red iron oxide
1 drop ultramarine blue

1. Combine the foundation base and yellow iron oxide in your mixing container.

2. Blend mechanically for 1 minute.

3. Add the remaining ingredients on the list, blending for 1 minute after each addition.

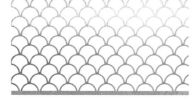

LOOKS GREAT WITH

Skin undertone: Cool and
  neutral

Other uses: Eye shadow

SUGAR COOKIE

This creamy-looking medium beige foundation can double as a matte eye shadow.

2 teaspoons any white foundation base (pages 135–141)

1 teaspoon any yellow foundation base, made by substituting yellow iron oxide for titanium dioxide and/or zinc oxide in any of the foundation base recipes (pages 135–141)

½ teaspoon titanium dioxide

1 smidgen plus 1 drop yellow iron oxide

1 drop red iron oxide

1 drop ultramarine blue

1. Combine the white and yellow foundation bases in your mixing container.

2. Blend mechanically for 1 minute.

3. Add the remaining ingredients on the list, blending for 1 minute after each addition.

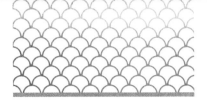

LOOKS GREAT WITH
Skin undertone: Neutral
Other uses: Eye shadow, blush,
bronzer

CAKE

The light beige tones in this foundation make it a subtle matte tan eye shadow, too.

1½ teaspoons any yellow foundation base, made by substituting yellow iron oxide for titanium dioxide and/or zinc oxide in any of the foundation base recipes (pages 135–141)

1 teaspoon any white foundation base (pages 135–141)

1 smidgen red iron oxide

1 smidgen ultramarine blue

1 smidgen yellow iron oxide

1. Combine the yellow and white foundation bases in your mixing container.

2. Blend mechanically for 1 minute.

3. Add the remaining ingredients on the list, blending for 1 minute after each addition.

Veronica is wearing

EYES: Cashmere, Briar, and Lilac shadows; Fern Gully eyeliner

LIPS: Basic Lip Gloss mixed with Sugar Peach

FACE: Cake foundation; Suede bronzer; Cherry Blossom blush; Wonderland highlighter

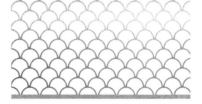

CREAM PUFF

The medium golden-tan tones in this foundation also work well as
a light brown matte eye shadow.

2½ teaspoons any white foundation
base (pages 135–141)

½ teaspoon plus 1 smidgen yellow
iron oxide

1 tad titanium dioxide

1 smidgen plus 1 drop red iron
oxide

1 smidgen plus 1 drop ultramarine
blue

1. Combine the foundation base and yellow
iron oxide in your mixing container.

2. Blend mechanically for 1 minute.

3. Add the remaining ingredients on
the list, blending for 1 minute after
each addition.

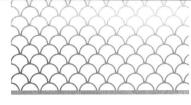

LOOKS GREAT WITH

Skin undertone: Warm

Other uses: Eye shadow,
bronzer

NUTMEG

This rich sandstone foundation looks perfect on the warm skin undertones common throughout Mediterranean and Latin American countries. It makes a lovely bronzer for those with lighter skin tones and can also be used as a matte eyeshadow.

2½ teaspoons any yellow foundation base, made by substituting yellow iron oxide for titanium dioxide and/or zinc oxide in any of the foundation base recipes (pages 135–141)

1 smidgen red iron oxide

1 smidgen ultramarine blue

1. Combine the foundation base and red iron oxide in your mixing container.

2. Blend mechanically for 1 minute.

3. Add the ultramarine blue and blend for 1 minute.

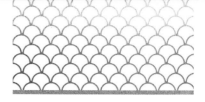

LOOKS GREAT WITH
Skin undertone: Warm
Other uses: Eye shadow,
   eyebrow powder, blush,
   bronzer

CINNAMON

This reddish-brown foundation also makes a beautifully warm matte brown eye shadow.

2½ teaspoons any yellow foundation base, made by substituting yellow iron oxide for titanium dioxide and/or zinc oxide in any of the foundation base recipes (pages 135–141)

1 tad yellow iron oxide

1 dash red iron oxide

1 pinch black iron oxide

1 pinch ultramarine blue

1. Combine the foundation base and yellow iron oxide in your mixing container.

2. Blend mechanically for 1 minute.

3. Add the remaining ingredients on the list, blending for 1 minute after each addition.

BROWN SUGAR

This creamy brown foundation can also be used as a dark brown matte eye shadow.

2½ teaspoons any yellow foundation base, made by substituting
   yellow iron oxide for titanium
   dioxide and/or zinc oxide in any
   of the foundation base recipes
   (pages 135–141)

½ teaspoon plus 1 dash yellow iron
   oxide

1 tad black iron oxide

1 tad red iron oxide

1 tad ultramarine blue

1. Combine the foundation base and yellow iron oxide in your mixing container.

2. Blend mechanically for 1 minute.

3. Add the remaining ingredients on the list, blending for 1 minute after each addition.

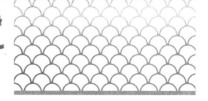

LOOKS GREAT WITH

Skin undertone: Warm
Other uses: Eye shadow,
   eyeliner, eyebrow powder,
   blush, bronzer

CARAMEL

This dark golden-brown foundation can be used as a medium brown matte eye shadow.

2½ teaspoons any yellow foundation base, made by substituting
   yellow iron oxide for titanium
   dioxide and/or zinc oxide in any
   of the foundation base recipes
   (pages 135–141)
1 tad plus 1 pinch yellow iron oxide
1 tad ultramarine blue
1 dash plus 1 pinch red iron oxide
1 pinch plus 1 smidgen black iron
   oxide

1. Combine the foundation base and yellow iron oxide in your mixing container.

2. Blend mechanically for 1 minute.

3. Add the remaining ingredients on the list, blending for 1 minute after each addition.

Sahira is wearing

EYES: Morgan le Fay and Sequins shadows; Fireflies eyeliner; Brunette eyebrow powder

LIPS: Basic Lip Gloss mixed with salmon mica

FACE: Caramel foundation; Vamp blush

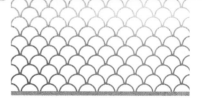

LOOKS GREAT WITH

Skin undertone: Cool and
neutral

Other uses: Eye shadow,
eyeliner, eyebrow powder,
bronzer

MILK CHOCOLATE

The deep reddish-brown tones in this foundation can do double
duty as a dark brown matte eye shadow.

2¹⁄₂ teaspoons any yellow foundation base, made by substituting
yellow iron oxide for titanium
dioxide and/or zinc oxide in any
of the foundation base recipes
(pages 135–141)

1 tad yellow iron oxide

1 dash plus 1 pinch black iron
oxide

1 dash plus 1 pinch ultramarine
blue

1 dash red iron oxide

1. Combine the foundation base and yellow
iron oxide in your mixing container.

2. Blend mechanically for 1 minute.

3. Add the remaining ingredients on
the list, blending for 1 minute after
each addition.

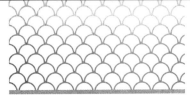

LOOKS GREAT WITH

Skin undertone: Neutral
Other uses: Eye shadow,
  eyeliner, eyebrow powder,
  bronzer

ROOT BEER

This is the darkest brown foundation recipe in this book. It also
makes a rich matte eye shadow.

2½ teaspoons any yellow foundation base, made by substituting
  yellow iron oxide for titanium
  dioxide and/or zinc oxide in any
  of the foundation base recipes
  (pages 135–141)
½ teaspoon plus 1 dash black iron
  oxide
½ teaspoon plus 1 dash ultramarine
  blue
1 tad plus 1 dash yellow iron oxide
1 tad red iron oxide

1. Combine the foundation base and black
   iron oxide in your mixing container.

2. Blend mechanically for 1 minute.

3. Add the remaining ingredients on
   the list, blending for 1 minute after
   each addition.

CONCEALERS

Having clear skin is important to me, so there is hardly a day I go without using concealer. Although the bad acne I used to have has cleared up since I started using my handmade makeup, my face still shows signs of scarring, redness, and uneven coloring, plus I have dark under-eye circles.

You can use foundation as a concealer, applying it with a damp brush to get even more coverage, or use the recipes that follow. See page 206 for additional application tips.

Each of the concealer recipes in the following section makes enough to fill one 10-gram jar.

PRO TIP

CONCEALER COLORS

The concealers shown on the facing page are only two of the colors that you can create. To ensure that your concealer has the same undertone and shade as your foundation, use your finished foundation as your base in the concealer recipes that follow.

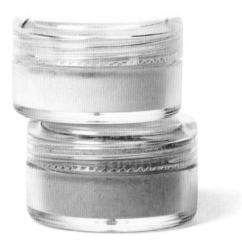

Other uses: Eye shadow

LIGHT CONCEALER

This light concealer is perfect for light to medium skin, regardless of undertone. Make it with the same foundation you wear. The concealer shown here was made with Sugar Cookie.

1 teaspoon finished light foundation of your choice (Vanilla, Eggnog, Sugar Cookie, Cake, Cream Puff, or Nutmeg, pages 143–149)

1 tad titanium dioxide

1. Combine the foundation and titanium dioxide in your mixing container.

2. Blend mechanically for 30 seconds.

Other uses: Eye shadow

DARK CONCEALER

This dark concealer is great for medium to dark skin colors and all undertones. Make it with the same foundation you wear. The concealer shown here was made with Brown Sugar.

1 teaspoon finished dark foundation of your choice (Cinnamon, Brown Sugar, Caramel, Milk Chocolate, or Root Beer, pages 150–155)

1 tad yellow iron oxide

1. Combine the foundation and yellow iron oxide in your mixing container.

2. Blend mechanically for 30 seconds.

COLOR CORRECTORS

Concealer is great for covering most flaws, but for extreme cases of discoloration, you can also apply color correctors underneath your foundation and concealer. If you find that the colors in the recipes that follow are too intense, try adding less pigment or more titanium dioxide to your foundation powder. If you want a darker color corrector, add more pigment than the recipe calls for. Never use color correctors on the skin alone! They are meant to be layered beneath foundation and concealer. Each recipe produces a different pastel color that neutralizes unwanted coloration such as redness, under-eye darkness, and sallow skin.

Each of the color corrector recipes in the following section makes enough to fill one 10-gram jar.

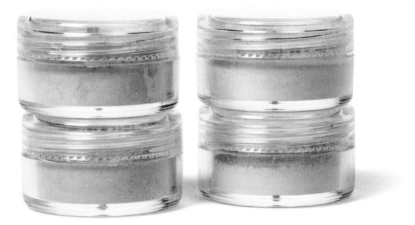

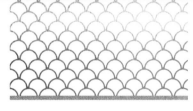

Other uses: Eye shadow

MINT COLOR CORRECTOR

Use this color corrector to camouflage acne and balance any pink or red discoloration caused by sensitive skin, scarring, rosacea, and even redness around the nostrils.

1 teaspoon Cream Puff foundation (page 148) or Simple Light Foundation Base (page 135)

½ teaspoon titanium dioxide

1 pinch chromium oxide green

1. Combine the foundation or foundation base and titanium dioxide in your mixing container.

2. Blend mechanically for 30 seconds.

3. Add the chromium oxide green and blend for 30 seconds.

Other uses: Eye shadow, eyebrow powder, foundation, blush

PEACH COLOR CORRECTOR

This color corrector balances dark under-eye circles for those with medium to dark skin, making tired eyes look brighter.

2 teaspoons Simple Dark Foundation Base (page 136)

1 tad plus 1 pinch yellow iron oxide

1 tad titanium dioxide

1 pinch plus 1 smidgen manganese violet

1 smidgen red iron oxide

1. Combine the foundation base and yellow iron oxide in your mixing container.

2. Blend mechanically for 30 seconds.

3. Add the remaining ingredients on the list, blending for 30 seconds after each addition.

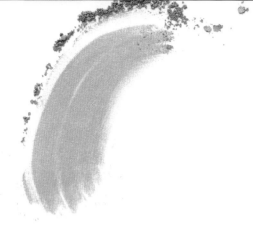

Other uses: Eye shadow

LILAC COLOR CORRECTOR

In addition to balancing sallow, yellow-looking skin, this color corrector can double as a subtle matte eye shadow.

1 teaspoon Cream Puff foundation (page 148) or Simple Light Foundation Base (page 135)

1 tad manganese violet

1 tad titanium dioxide

1 pinch ultramarine pink

1 smidgen ultramarine blue

1. Combine the foundation or foundation base and manganese violet in your mixing container.

2. Blend mechanically for 30 seconds.

3. Add the remaining ingredients on the list, blending for 30 seconds after each addition.

Other uses: Eye shadow

LEMON COLOR CORRECTOR

This color corrector counters the purple discoloration in dark under-eye circles. You can even add a little satin gold mica to give the corrector a bit of glow, which brightens your eyes and gives you an "awake" look.

½ teaspoon plus 1 tad Simple Dark Foundation Base (page 136)

1 tad yellow iron oxide

1 tad titanium dioxide

1. Combine the foundation base and yellow iron oxide in your mixing container.

2. Blend mechanically for 30 seconds.

3. Add the titanium dioxide and blend for 30 seconds.

SHIMMERY BLUSHES

These blushes add a pop of color to your cheeks, plus a little luster. If you have flawless skin, these blushes will draw attention to that and really brighten up your face. All of the recipes that follow can be used as a blush, lip color, and eye shadow. You can also mix these blushes together to create new shades. See page 206 for application tips.

Each of the shimmery blush recipes in the following section makes enough to fill one 30-gram jar.

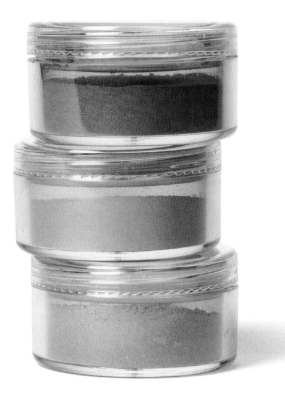

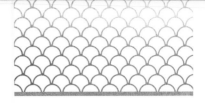

LOOKS GREAT WITH

Skin undertone: Neutral

Other uses: Eye shadow, lip color

VAMP

This is a deep-rose blush with a red glimmer.

1³⁄₄ teaspoons sericite
  1 tad Makeup Base (page 82 or 83)
¹⁄₂ teaspoon bright red mica
¹⁄₂ teaspoon satin sienna mica
  1 tad burgundy mica
  1 tad metallic gold mica
  1 tad satin beige mica

  Blend together using your preferred mixing method (page 66).

I love the makeup and style of the flappers and the early silver-screen sirens. For me, the word *vamp* always brings to mind black-and-white movies, layers of pearls and rhinestones, and thin overdrawn eyebrows and dark lips.

Lakshmi is wearing

EYES: Clancy and Peacock shadows; Peacock eyeliner; Fireflies eyebrow powder

LIPS: Basic Lip Gloss mixed with satin sienna mica

FACE: Honey foundation; Vamp blush

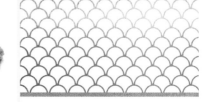

LOOKS GREAT WITH
Skin undertone: Warm and
　neutral
Other uses: Eye shadow,
　highlighter, lip color

SUGAR PEACH

This faint apricot blush has a gorgeous silver luster.

1½ teaspoons sericite
　1 tad Makeup Base (page 82 or 83)
¾ teaspoon salmon mica
　1 tad burgundy mica
　1 tad satin beige mica
　1 tad satin gold mica
　1 tad satin white mica

　Blend together using your preferred mixing method (page 66).

I call my daughters Sugar Peach and Sweet Pea. They are just so perfect and cute.

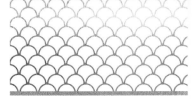

LOOKS GREAT WITH

Skin undertone: Warm

Other uses: Eye shadow,
highlighter, lip color

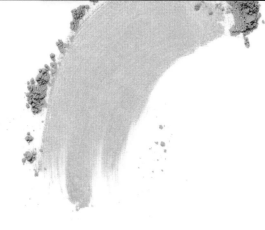

One of my favorite singers is
Gwen Stefani. Her Japanese
backup singers introduced me
to the youthful street style
known as *harajuku*.

HARAJUKU

This is a lovely sparkly dusty-pink blush.

1³/₄ teaspoons sericite

1 tad Makeup Base (page 82 or 83)

1¹/₂ teaspoons salmon mica

1 tad bright red mica

1 tad pink blue mica

1 tad satin gold mica

Blend together using your preferred mixing
method (page 66).

MATTE BLUSHES

Matte blushes look good on everyone but are especially flattering if you have acne or large pores. A good matte blush should be sheer enough to give your cheeks just a bit of color. These recipes give a faint flush while allowing the skin to shine through. All of them can be used as eye shadow. You can also mix any of these blushes together, or add in a bit of mica for some shine. See page 206 for application tips.

Each of the matte blush recipes in the following section makes enough to fill one 30-gram jar.

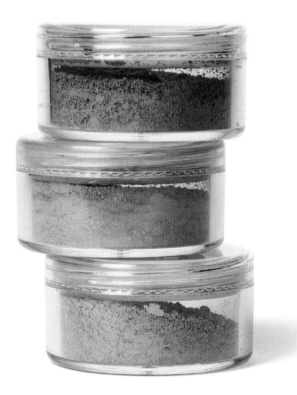

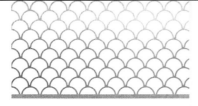

LOOKS GREAT WITH

Skin undertone: Cool and
neutral

Other uses: Eye shadow

We had a cherry blossom tree
outside my childhood home. I
remember lying underneath it
and watching as the wind blew
blossom petals down like con-
fetti. It was one of the prettiest
things I have ever seen.

CHERRY BLOSSOM

This is a neutral dusty-rose blush.

1³/4 teaspoons sericite
1 tad Makeup Base (page 82 or 83)
1 pinch red iron oxide
1 pinch titanium dioxide
1 smidgen ultramarine blue

1. Combine the sericite and Makeup Base in
   your mixing container.

2. Blend mechanically for 1 minute.

3. Add the remaining ingredients on the list,
   blending for 1 minute after each addition.

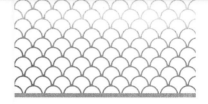

LOOKS GREAT WITH
Skin undertone: Warm
Other uses: Eye shadow

CORAL

This blush is the perfect peachy tone.

1³/₄ teaspoons sericite
 ¹/₂ teaspoon titanium dioxide
   1 tad plus 1 pinch yellow iron oxide
   1 tad Makeup Base (page 82 or 83)
   1 dash plus 1 pinch red iron oxide

1. Combine the sericite and titanium dioxide in your mixing container.

2. Blend mechanically for 1 minute.

3. Adding the remaining ingredients on the list, blending for 1 minute after each addition.

Coral is one of my favorite colors, and it is flattering on everyone.

Carly is wearing

EYES: Sequins, Morgan le Fay, and Nectar shadows; Peacock eyeliner

LIPS: Basic Lip Gloss mixed with Vamp

FACE: Cake and Honey foundations; Coral blush; Heatherbelle highlighter

LOOKS GREAT WITH
Skin undertone: Neutral
Other uses: Eye shadow

CUPCAKE

This powdery blush is baby-doll pink.

1³/4 teaspoon sericite
 1 tad Makeup Base (page 82 or 83)
 1 tad titanium dioxide
 1 pinch red iron oxide
 1 pinch ultramarine pink

1. Combine the sericite and Makeup Base in your mixing container.

2. Blend mechanically for 1 minute.

3. Add the remaining ingredients on the list, blending for 1 minute after each addition.

I once worked in a cupcake bakery with a girl who was one of the most original, pink, glittery, and cartoonlike people I have ever known. She made every day at work fun and entertaining. This color reminds me of her.

SHIMMERY BRONZERS

Bronzers are beautiful all year round. In the summer, they draw attention to your glowing skin. In the winter, they add a bit of color. I like pearlescent bronzers for tan and darker skin colors and matte bronzers for pale and light skin colors. But the choice is up to you! See page 207 for application tips.

Each of the shimmery bronzer recipes in the following section makes enough to fill one 30-gram jar.

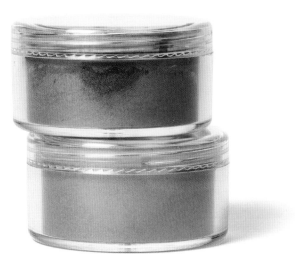

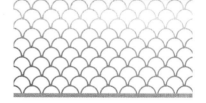

LOOKS GREAT WITH

Skin undertone: Cool and
neutral

Other uses: Eye shadow,
eyeliner, lip color

TOFFEE

This lustrous milk-chocolate bronzer can also be used as a medium
brown eye shadow.

1 tad sericite

1 dash Makeup Base (page 82
or 83)

3/4 teaspoon smoky gold mica

1 tad plus 1 dash satin bronze mica

1 tad plus 1 dash satin gold mica

Blend together using your preferred
mixing method (page 66).

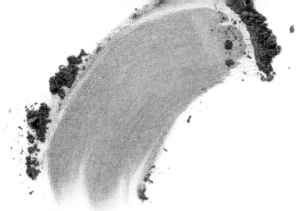

LOOKS GREAT WITH

Skin undertone: Warm

Other uses: Eye shadow,
  eyeliner, highlighter, lip
  color

SUN-KISSED

This sparkly copper-gold highlighter also makes a beautiful medium golden-brown eye shadow.

- 1 tad sericite
- 1 dash Makeup Base (page 82 or 83)
- 1 tad plus 1 dash metallic gold mica
- 1 tad plus 1 dash metallic orange mica
- 1 tad mica satin bronze mica
- 1 tad satin gold mica
- 1 dash smoky gold mica

Blend together using your preferred mixing method (page 66).

MATTE BRONZERS

Matte bronzers are great for lighter skin colors or for contouring the face. For the most natural bronzer, you can use your unique foundation color blend, then make it just a bit darker by adding a mixture of yellow, red, and black iron oxides. To make the following matte bronzers shimmer, feel free to add a little mica! See page 207 for application tips.

Each of the matte bronzer recipes in the following section makes enough to fill one 30-gram jar.

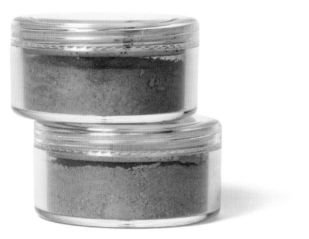

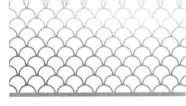

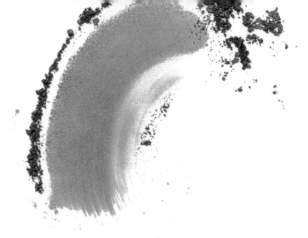

SUEDE

The cool cinnamon-brown tones in this bronzer make it a beautiful medium brown eye shadow or blush for medium skin colors. It also works well as an eyebrow powder for blondes and brunettes.

1 teaspoon sericite

3/4 teaspoon yellow iron oxide

1 dash Makeup Base (page 82 or 83)

1 pinch plus 1 smidgen ultramarine blue

1 smidgen black iron oxide

1 pinch red iron oxide

1 smidgen titanium dioxide

1. Combine the sericite and yellow iron oxide in your mixing container.

2. Blend mechanically for 1 minute.

3. Add the remaining ingredients on the list, blending for 1 minute after each addition.

LOOKS GREAT WITH
Skin undertone: Warm
Other uses: Eye shadow,
    eyeliner, eyebrow powder,
    foundation, blush

HONEY

This golden–medium brown bronzer makes a great eyebrow powder for blondes and brunettes. You can also use it as a matte eye shadow or a blush for medium to dark skin.

1 teaspoon sericite
1 tad yellow iron oxide
1 dash Makeup Base (page 82 or 83)
1 pinch red iron oxide
1 smidgen black iron oxide

1. Combine the sericite and yellow iron oxide in your mixing container.

2. Blend mechanically for 1 minute.

3. Add the remaining ingredients on the list, blending for 1 minute after each addition.

Lucy is wearing

EYES: Calgary shadow; Peacock eyeliner; Oak eyebrow powder

LIPS: Basic Lip Gloss mixed with satin copper mica

FACE: Cake foundation; Honey bronzer; Coral blush; Bombshell highlighter

FINISHING POWDER

Finishing powder helps set liquid and cream makeup and eliminates shiny skin. If you have oily skin, try using finishing powder throughout the day to keep your face looking flawlessly matte. Many different ingredients can be used to create an effective finishing powder, including rice powder, cornstarch, kaolin, and silica. For the simplest of options, try using 100 percent rice powder.

3   **tads plus 1 dash rice powder**
3   **tads plus 1 dash sericite**
1   **dash Makeup Base (page 82 or 83)**
3   **tads plus 1 dash silica**

Yield: 1 (30-gram) jar

1. Combine all the ingredients except silica in your mixing container.

2. Blend mechanically for 4 minutes.

3. Incorporate the silica by hand with your preferred mixing method (page 66).

VARIATIONS

What follows are ideas for how to create a finishing powder that is perfect for your skin and your needs. Use the main recipe as a guide for quantities, and then substitute the ingredients I suggest. Play around with quantities of your substitutions to make a powder that feels and looks great!

▶ Those in the entertainment industry will benefit from adding silica powder, which helps make the skin look flawless in photographs and even in high-definition TV.

▶ For an extremely silky and sheer botanical alternative, use tapioca starch and arrowroot powder.

▶ If you have oily and/or acne-prone skin, make your finishing powder with kaolin, silica, or calcium carbonate to help regulate excess oil.

▶ Try a mixture of rice power and allantoin for a healing version.

▶ For a slightly tinted alternative, add a small amount of your foundation or some iron oxides and ultramarine blue to your finishing powder.

▶ Finally, to create a finishing powder with a slight shimmer, add some satin white mica.

If you have dry skin or like cream and liquid makeup products, try this mixing medium. You can add it to any powder mineral makeup to turn it into a liquid or cream. This mixing medium can also be used on its own as a setting spray to help your makeup last throughout the day. Or apply it as a skin refresher: instead of touching up your makeup later in the day, just spray a little mixing medium on your face, blot with a tissue, and you're good to go!

3 **parts distilled water**
1 **part glycerin**

1. Measure the water and glycerin into a spray bottle with a fine mist and mix thoroughly.

2. Pour into a clean dish some of the powder makeup you want to use as a cream or liquid. Spray a small amount of the mixing medium into the dish and combine with a makeup brush. The more mixing medium you add, the more liquid the makeup will be.

PRO TIP
SHAKE IT OUT
To avoid the spread of bacteria, never put any water or mixing medium directly into your jar of makeup. Instead, shake out some powder into the jar's lid or onto the back of your hand, then add water.

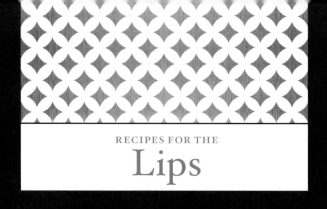

Lips

The color you choose to wear on your lips can completely change your look. Darkly colored lips are amazing for a night on the town but can seem overdone for daytime wear. Bright colors draw the eye's attention and work best on big lips, whereas paler tones provide a flattering everyday effect on both small and large lips. You can make either statement by adding color to the basic lip balm and lip gloss recipes that follow.

First you'll need to decide what kind of product you want to wear. Lip balm is usually clear but can come in lightly tinted shades. Lip gloss is usually colored, serving as a more casual and moisturizing choice than lipstick.

There are two simple ways you can add color to the Firm Lip Balm (page 184), Moisturizing Lip Balm (page 186), or Basic Lip Gloss (page 188) recipes: mix in

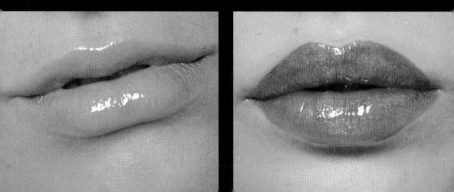

pure mica for a sparkly but sheer effect or — to create a more opaque product — blend in matte pigment and titanium dioxide or one of the eye or face recipes I suggest for use on the lips. Whichever method you choose, make sure the colors you add are approved for use on the lips (see Color Me Safe, page 189).

In the lip recipes that follow, I include some moisturizing ingredients like waxes and oils. The ones I use have long shelf lives: beeswax lasts indefinitely, while jojoba oil should last for five years if stored properly. When you make your products, you have many substitution options, including candelilla, carnauba, or soy wax, and almond, avocado, or olive oil, to name just a few. If you decide to use a different oil or wax than what's called for in the recipe, though, be sure to look at the new ingredient's shelf life. Your finished product will last only as long as the shortest shelf life of your ingredients. For example, if you use rose hip seed oil, your finished product can go rancid after six months.

LIP BALMS AND GLOSSES

These lip balm and lip gloss recipes are easy and versatile. If you want your lips to have a hint of color, you can add micas. If you want to add some flavoring — such as lavender essential oil — you can! Just follow the directions on the label of whatever you add, paying attention to the suggested amounts of flavoring.

PRO TIP
HEATING INGREDIENTS
When making lip gloss and lip balm, you will need to heat ingredients such as coconut oil and beeswax that are solid at room temperature.

Always cut the solid oils and waxes into small pieces and heat them slowly to prevent the final product from becoming brittle.

Never microwave or heat dry iron oxides or pigments, as they can light on fire. If you need to microwave a product with iron oxide or pigments in it, fully mix the concoction and make sure the pigments are thoroughly wet.

FIRM LIP BALM

This is the easiest lip balm recipe ever! All you need is a little oil and wax. It is somewhat sturdier than the Moisturizing Lip Balm (page 186). Due to its stiffness, this lip balm can be difficult to apply with a finger, but it works well in a tube. It offers the perfect amount of moisture in the winter or any time you have chapped lips.

1½   **teaspoons beeswax
        granules or shredded
        beeswax**
4½   **teaspoons jojoba oil**

Yield: 4 (4-gram) tubes

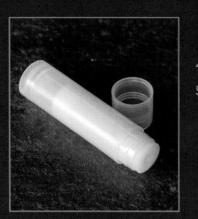

1. Place the wax in a microwavable bowl or in a pot for stovetop heating.

2. Add the oil and slowly heat until the wax is liquid, stirring every few seconds.

3. Carefully transfer the hot liquid into lip balm tubes using a syringe. Work quickly to prevent the mixture from cooling and solidifying before you have finished.

4. Let cool for about 20 minutes.

5. Use a flat scraper or knife to cut the balm level with the tops of the lip balm tubes, then cap the tubes.

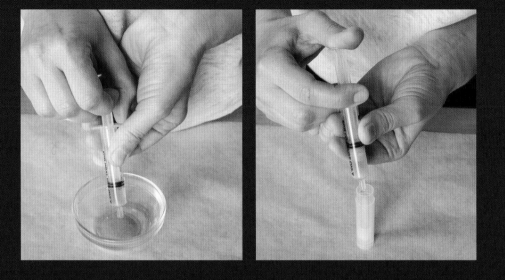

PRO TIP
TROUBLESHOOTING LIP BALM

PROBLEM	SOLUTION
Too hard	Add more oils.
Too soft	Add more wax.
Too sheer	Add more pigments.
Too opaque	Add more oils.
Lip balm breaks off	Wind the tube up as far as it will go, cut off the lip balm, melt it, and quickly refill the tube before the mixture cools.

MOISTURIZING LIP BALM

This lip balm is soft and supple. It would even make a great salve for very dry skin: you can use it on your hands, feet, and elbows! Store it in a small jar or metal tin, and apply with a finger or lip brush.

- 1 teaspoon jojoba oil
- 1 tad any lip-safe mica(s) (optional)
- 1–2 smidgens any lip-safe oxide(s) (optional)
- 1 teaspoon beeswax granules or shredded beeswax
- 1 teaspoon coconut oil
- ½ teaspoon cocoa butter

Yield: 3–4 (10-gram) jars

1. Combine the jojoba oil with the mica(s) and oxide(s), if using, and stir until thoroughly mixed, with no streaks.

2. Combine the beeswax, coconut oil, and cocoa butter in a heatproof container. Heat slowly in a microwave or on the stovetop until melted, stirring often.

3. Stir the pigment-and-oil mixture into the melted solids until fully combined, with no streaks.

4. Slowly pour the hot liquid mixture into jars, leaving enough room for the lids to be screwed on.

5. Let cool for about 20 minutes, then screw on the lids.

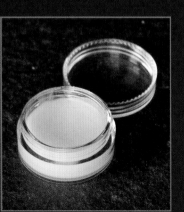

Janel is wearing

EYES: Morgan Le Fay shadow; Sun-Kissed eyeliner

LIPS: Basic Lip Gloss mixed with Coral

FACE: Eggnog foundation; Honey bronzer; Cupcake blush; Nectar highlighter

BASIC LIP GLOSS

You can create your own simple lip gloss by mixing micas and/or pigments with castor oil and another oil. Using castor oil alone can dry out the lips, so it is important to include an additional fat. In the recipe below, that is the Moisturizing Lip Balm Base.

For a very subtle shimmer of color add any lip-safe mica. Pigments will result in a more opaque product and are a great option if you want a bright, dark, or intense lip gloss. Including both mica and pigment will create bright, bold colors with some glimmer. Another option for adding color is to mix in any of my lip-safe eye or face products. See page 209 for application tips.

20 milliliters castor oil

1 tad any lip-safe mica(s) (optional)

1 dash any lip-safe pigment(s) (optional)

½ teaspoon Moisturizing Lip Balm (page 186)

Yield: 1 (¼-fluid-ounce) tube

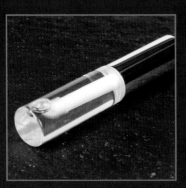

1. Combine the castor oil with the mica(s) and pigment(s), if using, and stir until thoroughly mixed, with no streaks.

2. Measure out the lip balm into a heatproof container. Heat slowly in a microwave or on the stovetop until melted, stirring often.

3. Stir the pigment-and-oil mixture into the melted lip balm base until fully combined, with no streaks.

4. Stand the lip gloss tube upright, then pour in the liquid using a plastic syringe or metal flavor injector. Fill to the rim, insert the lip gloss wand, and screw the lid on tight.

TROUBLESHOOTING LIP GLOSS

PROBLEM	SOLUTION
Lid won't close properly	Use an empty syringe to suck out excess liquid.
Marbling	Add pigment to the oil first, then add to the melted balm.
Lumpy	Continue mixing.

COLOR ME SAFE

Before you add any color to your lip balm or gloss, make sure that color is safe to use on your lips. This list is a good place to start, but always double-check ingredients on the FDA's website.

LIP-SAFE

» Black iron oxide
» Bright red
» Burgundy
» Glimmering brown blue
» Glimmering white
» Manganese violet
» Metallic gold
» Metallic olive
» Metallic orange
» Muted gold
» Muted silver
» Pale yellow green
» Peach gold
» Pink blue
» Red iron oxide
» Salmon
» Satin beige
» Satin black
» Satin bronze
» Satin brown blue
» Satin copper
» Satin gold
» Satin sienna
» Satin white
» Silver gold
» Smoky blue
» Smoky gold
» Smoky green
» Titanium dioxide
» White gold
» Yellow iron oxide

NOT LIP-SAFE

» Chromium oxide green
» Hydrated chromium oxide green
» Nude silver
» Ultramarine blue
» Ultramarine pink
» Ultramarine violet

Micas are indicated in green. Matte pigments are in pink.

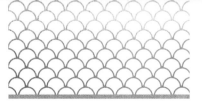

LOOKS GREAT WITH
Skin undertone: Neutral

RUBY RED

This lip gloss is perfect for a night on the town. Combine with winged eyeliner and false eyelashes for a fabulous pinup girl look.

20 milliliters castor oil
½ teaspoon bright red mica
1 smidgen red iron oxide
½ teaspoon Moisturizing Lip Balm (page 186)

Yield: 1 (¼-fluid-ounce) tube

1. Combine the castor oil with the mica. Stir until thoroughly mixed, with no streaks.

2. Add the oxide and stir until thoroughly mixed, with no streaks.

3. Measure out the lip balm base into a heatproof container. Heat slowly in a microwave or on the stovetop until melted, stirring often.

4. Stir the mica-and-oil mixture into the melted lip balm base until fully combined, with no streaks.

5. Stand the lip gloss tube upright, then pour in the liquid using a plastic syringe or metal flavor injector. Fill to the rim, insert the lip gloss wand, and screw the lid on tight.

Nani is wearing

EYES: Buttercream shadow; Fireflies eyeliner

LIPS: Ruby Red, with Flurries in the center

FACE: Nutmeg–Cream Puff foundation mixture (50:50); Suede bronzer; Vamp blush; Flurries highlighter

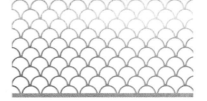

LOOKS GREAT WITH
Skin undertone: Cool and
neutral

FOXY

This is a shimmery nude copper with hints of metallic silver that makes a gorgeous summer lip color for bronzed skin.

20 milliliters castor oil
1 pinch pale yellow green mica
1 pinch peach gold mica
1 pinch salmon mica
1 pinch satin beige mica
1 pinch satin brown blue mica
1 pinch satin white mica
½ teaspoon Moisturizing Lip Balm (page 186)

Yield: 1 (¼-fluid-ounce) bottle

1. Combine the castor oil with all of the micas. Stir until thoroughly mixed, with no streaks.

2. Measure out the lip balm base into a heatproof container. Heat slowly in a microwave or on the stovetop until melted, stirring often.

3. Stir the mica-and-oil mixture into the melted lip balm base until fully combined, with no streaks.

4. Stand the lip gloss tube upright, then pour in the liquid using a plastic syringe or metal flavor injector. Fill to the rim, insert the lip gloss wand, and screw the lid on tight.

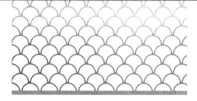

Skin undertone: Warm

ORANGE SHERBET

This pastel peach-orange lip gloss is perfect when paired with dark, smoky eye shadow. Its pale color is also fabulous for a 1960s mod makeup look.

20 milliliters castor oil

1 tad titanium dioxide

1 pinch yellow iron oxide

1 smidgen red iron oxide

1 pinch plus 1 smidgen peach gold mica

1 pinch plus 1 smidgen salmon mica

1 pinch pink blue mica

1 pinch silver gold mica

1/2 teaspoon Moisturizing Lip Balm (page 186)

Yield: 1 (¼-fluid-ounce) bottle

1. Combine the castor oil with the titanium dioxide and yellow and red iron oxides. Mix with a small whisk until fully combined.

2. Add all of the micas to the oil-oxide mixture and stir until there are no lumps.

3. Measure out the lip balm base into a heatproof container. Heat slowly in a microwave or on the stovetop until melted, stirring often.

4. Stir the colored oil mixture into the melted lip balm base until fully combined, with no streaks.

5. Stand the lip gloss tube upright, then pour in the liquid using a plastic syringe or metal flavor injector. Fill to the rim, insert the lip gloss wand, and screw the lid on tight.

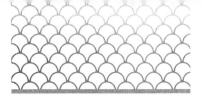

GIRL CRUSH

This lustrous nude golden-apricot lip gloss looks great day or night. Pair it with a pearlescent bronzer and pale eye shadow for a day look, or with dark eyeliner and smoky eye shadow for a night look.

20 milliliters castor oil
 1 pinch plus 1 smidgen glimmering white mica
 1 pinch plus 1 smidgen peach gold mica
 1 pinch plus 1 smidgen salmon mica
 1 pinch plus 1 smidgen satin beige mica
 1 pinch satin copper mica
 ½ teaspoon Moisturizing Lip Balm (page 186)

Yield: 1 (¼-fluid-ounce) bottle

1. Combine the castor oil with the micas. Stir until thoroughly mixed, with no streaks.

2. Measure out the lip balm base into a heatproof container. Heat slowly in a microwave or on the stovetop until melted, stirring often.

3. Stir the mica-and-oil mixture into the melted lip balm base until fully combined, with no streaks.

4. Stand the lip gloss tube upright, then pour in the liquid using a plastic syringe or metal flavor injector. Fill to the rim, insert the lip gloss wand, and screw the lid on tight.

Germaine is wearing

EYES: Kitty-Cat, Nectar, and Heatherbelle shadows; Bonsai eyeliner

FACE: Eggnog foundation; Suede bronzer; Coral blush; Heatherbelle highlighter

LIPS: Girl Crush

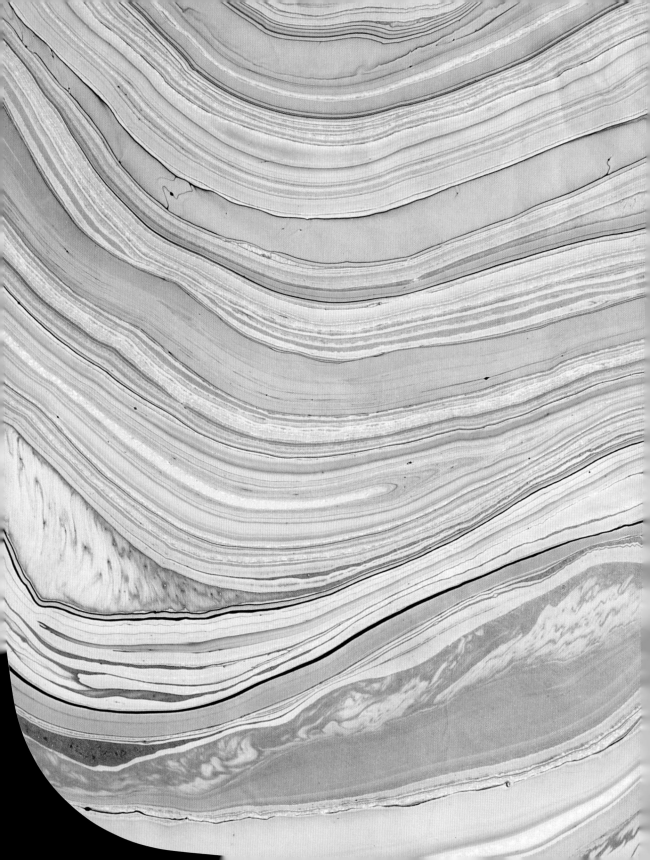

CHAPTER 7

LET'S PUT IT ON

When I was a kid I sought beauty in perfection. As I got older I began to value the imperfect — for it is there that the unique, the authentic is manifest. It is there that we see that which makes us an individual and unique.

SUSAN SARANDON

Now that you've created some makeup, surely you are eager to test it out. Before you do, it is important to understand that the structure of mineral makeup is different from that of the cosmetics you buy commercially, and that fact affects its application. Mineral makeup has fewer ingredients and is more pigmented than most store-bought cosmetics. A little mineral makeup goes a long way! Be sure to blend, blend, blend. Start with a light layer, only adding more if you need extra coverage. If you find the makeup is too concentrated, you can add some sericite to make it subtler and easier to apply.

You can also experiment with applying mineral makeup in different states: use the makeup wet or dry, or mix it with sunscreens, lotions, serum, or any other mixing medium. To apply your mineral makeup wet, first pour some powder into a lid or onto the back of your hand, then either use a damp brush to apply the makeup, or use a brush to mix the powder with some water or mixing medium and then apply. If you want lighter coverage, add a dash of foundation to your regular face lotion. The more powder you add, the more coverage the makeup will offer, while the less powder you use, the more transluscent your coverage will be.

To ensure your makeup stays free of bacteria, mix up only enough liquid and makeup for one use, then throw away leftovers. Never add liquid of any kind directly to your container of powdered makeup.

A BRUSH BY ANY NAME

Even the most beautiful makeup won't look flawless if it is applied with the wrong tools. Mineral makeup powders apply best with brushes that have natural — rather than synthetic — bristles. If you decide to turn your makeup into a liquid form, however, synthetic brushes will give you a smoother application than natural bristles. For the best results, make sure your skin is always clean and moisturized, and have on hand a variety of clean, high-quality brushes, including:

- ▸ A kabuki brush to apply foundation dry
- ▸ A fluffy blush brush
- ▸ An eye shadow brush for applying and blending
- ▸ An angled brush to apply eyeliner and eyebrow powder

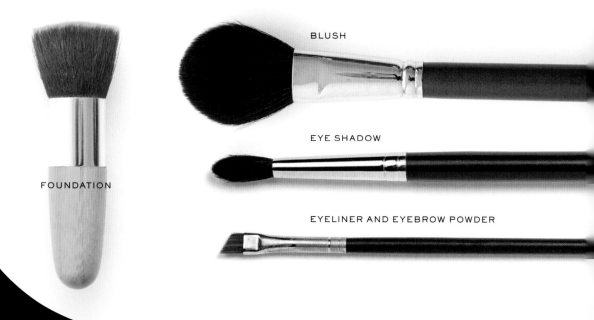

FOUNDATION

BLUSH

EYE SHADOW

EYELINER AND EYEBROW POWDER

Wash the brushes you use at home weekly. Set out a clean, dry towel and fill a bowl or sink with hot water. Dip the bristles of each brush into the water. Be sure not to soak the whole brush, as this can loosen the glue under the metal band, which holds the bristles in place. Place a small drop of facial soap into the palm of your hand or onto a clean plate, then gently rub the brush bristles back and forth and in a circular motion until all the bristles are covered in soap and some makeup product comes out of the brush. Rinse the brush, then continue the cycle of rinsing, washing with soap, and rinsing again, until the bristles are clean and the water runs clear. If you are applying makeup on other people, spot-clean your brushes with a disinfecting brush spray after each person.

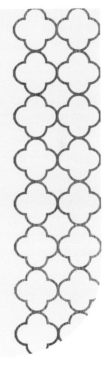

BEAUTY SPOT
SAFE USE AND APPLICATION

Always use your cosmetics as directed and make sure you are following any restrictions that might be relevant to individual ingredients. To keep yourself safe and your skin healthy, follow these tips when using makeup:

TEST THE PRODUCT on a small part of your jawline for one hour before applying it to a larger, and possibly more sensitive, area on your face to see if your skin has any negative reactions.

USE A CLEAN COTTON SWAB each time you sample a new pigment or finished makeup. Never use your fingers!

NEVER SHARE your cosmetics with anyone.

NOTE THE EXPIRATION DATE of each item and/or ingredient, and discard it when it has expired. Also, if your makeup ever changes color, texture, or smell, throw it out!

FACE AND EYE SHAPES

Note the shape of your face and eyes. Most makeup artists believe the ideal face shape is oval, since that well-balanced proportion is pleasing to the eye. But by using blush, bronzer, contour, and highlighter, you can learn how to best frame your face shape, helping your natural beauty shine through. Eye shadow application and color can also visually alter eye shape.

HOW TO APPLY

There are many ways to put on your makeup. Don't be afraid to play around and come up with a method that works best for you. I like to start with a clean face, then add a primer or facial lotion to even out my skin texture and help my makeup last all day. Then I work in any color correctors if needed, following up by addressing my eyes. I then apply foundation and concealer, followed by bronzer, blush, and highlighter, saving the lips for last.

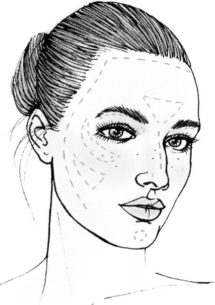

One method for applying bronzer, highlighter, and blush

BRONZER

BLUSH

HIGHLIGHTER

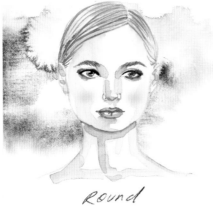

Round

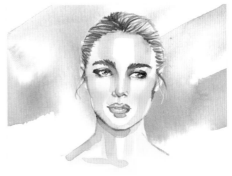

Oval

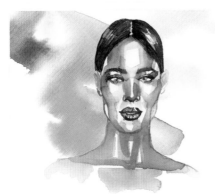

Long

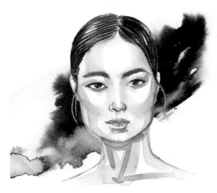

Square

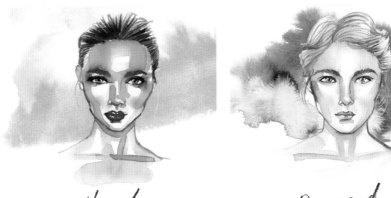

Heart

Diamond

Eye Shadow

One of the most common questions I get is how to apply eye shadow. This is tricky, because there really isn't one single right way to apply it. There are hundreds of options, depending on your eye shape, personal style preferences, and the occasion. That range of options can be either liberating or overwhelming. Here I explain two basic looks, and from there you can experiment with more advanced techniques.

DAY LOOK

Choose two colors. One should be a medium neutral color (such as tan, brown, gray, blue, or even a muted non-neutral tone) and the other should be a lighter highlight (such as white, cream, or even baby pink).

1. Using a damp angled eyeliner brush, apply your highlight color to the bone just beneath your eyebrow and to the inner corners of your eyelid. If you have close-set eyes, apply more toward the middle eyelid instead of the inner corner.

2. Using a fluffy eye shadow blending brush or your fingertips, apply your medium neutral color all over your eyelid.

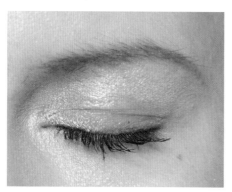

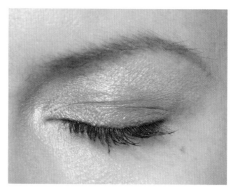

STEP 1 COLOR OPTIONS
Bombshell, Briar, Buttercream, Cream Soda, Fairy Floss, Flurries, Heatherbelle, Nectar, Vanilla, Wonderland

STEP 2 COLOR OPTIONS
Bambi, Beach Bunny, Cake, Calgary, Clancy, Cream Soda, Morgan le Fay, Nutmeg, Stargirl, Undine

Choose three monochromatic colors: a light, medium, and dark. The possibilities are endless. You could use white, gray, and black or cream, tan, and brown. Try smoky blues, plums, greens, or even bronze shades.

1. Using an eye shadow blending brush or your fingertips, apply your light color all over your eyelid and under your brow line.

   STEP 1 COLOR OPTIONS
   Bombshell, Buttercream, Fairy Floss, Flurries, Heatherbelle, Nectar, Vanilla, Wonderland

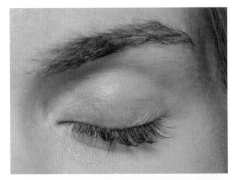

2. Using the same brush, apply your medium color focusing around the crease and outer half of your eyelid.

   STEP 2 COLOR OPTIONS
   Bambi, Beach Bunny, Bones, Cake, Cashmere, Clancy, Cream Soda, Fern Gully, Morgan le Fay, Nutmeg, Oak, Stargirl, Undine

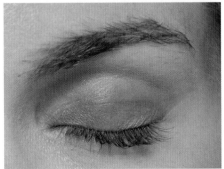

3. Using the same brush, apply the dark color from the outer corner of your eyelid to the crease. With a larger, fluffier brush, blend the dark color upward, toward your eyebrow.

   STEP 3 COLOR OPTIONS
   Bonsai, Brown Sugar, Calgary, Chimney, Echo, Fireflies, Kitty-Cat, Milk Chocolate, Peacock, Root Beer, Rueger, Sequins

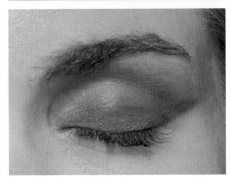

4. For a more dramatic look, you can extend that dark color below your eye, using your smaller eyeshadow brush, and complete the look with eyeliner applied to the upper lid.

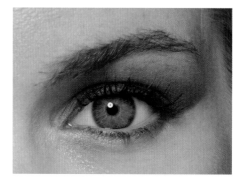

Eyeliner

Eyeliner can be applied either wet, for an intense sharp line, or dry, for a softer look. Use an angled brush for a thick, dramatic line or any other small eyeliner brush for just a hint of color.

To apply dry, use short, overlapping brushstrokes, starting in the inner corner of your eyelid and working toward the outer corner.

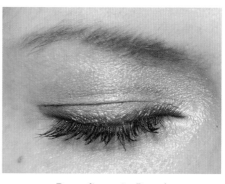

Dry eyeliner, using Peacock

To apply wet, dampen your brush with some mixing medium, then dip the brush into some loose powder, blending on the back of your hand before applying.

For a long-lasting eyeliner, first apply the color wet, then top it off with dry powder of the same color. Use two different colors to achieve a one-of-a-kind look: first apply a dark shade wet, then layer a lighter powder on top.

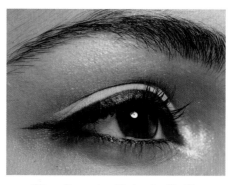

Wet eyeliner, winged look, using Fireflies

This popular look outlines the shape of the eye while extending and exaggerating the natural line of the top eyelashes. For best results, apply your eyeliner wet. If you plan to wear eye shadow, apply it before starting on your eyeliner.

1. Starting at the inner corner of your eye, draw a straight line following the edge of your eyelid.
2. Return to the center of this line and apply a second line, moving toward the outer corner of your eyelid and angling upward. The sharper the angle, the more dramatic your finished look will be. When you are done with this step, you will have two lines with some empty space in between toward the outer corner of your eye.
3. Fill in that space with eyeliner to complete the look.

Foundation

You can apply your foundation either wet or dry. A wet application will give you fuller coverage, while a dry application results in a lighter, sheerer look. Either way, avoid applying foundation around your eyes if you plan to use concealer; this will prevent the makeup around your eyes from becoming too thick.

WET FOUNDATION

Combine a dash of foundation with one or two sprays of mixing medium or a few drops of water — just enough liquid to create a creamy consistency. Apply it with a foundation brush or a blending sponge. Tap the brush or sponge into the foundation and start applying at the center of the face, blending outward. For a lighter look, mix your dry foundation with your normal face lotion, serum, or sunscreen, then apply with a synthetic foundation brush or clean hands.

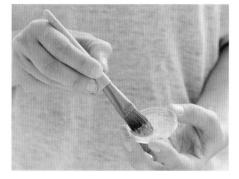

Blending dry foundation with mixing medium for a creamy consistency that offers heavier coverage.

DRY FOUNDATION

To apply your foundation dry, simply tap some powder into the lid of your foundation jar, swirl your brush in it, and tap off any excess powder. Then buff the foundation onto your skin using circular motions. To help smooth out the layer and avoid a powdery look, lightly spray a small amount of mixing medium (page 181) directly onto your face after applying the powder.

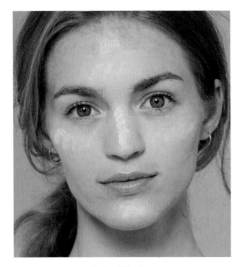

Before blending

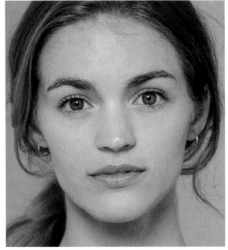

Dry foundation, using Eggnog

Concealer

To avoid powder settling into and drawing attention to fine wrinkles under your eyes, mix your concealer powder with moisturizer, eye cream, or serum before applying to dark under-eye circles. If you want to use concealer to camouflage dark under-eye circles, acne, scarring, or redness, you can apply it with either a damp or dry concealer brush. If you're applying it under your eyes, dot the concealer on your skin starting near your tear ducts and moving outward. Blend either by patting with your finger or dabbing with a sponge. You can then add some finishing powder on top of the concealer to set it.

Bronzer

For a sun-kissed look, apply bronzer using an angled bronzer brush anywhere on your face the sun would touch, including the top of your forehead, the tops of your cheeks (or the hollows of your cheeks for a contoured look), the tip of your nose, and your chin.

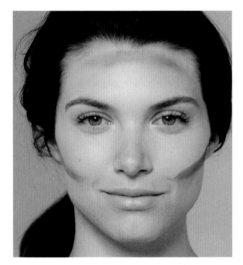

Before blending

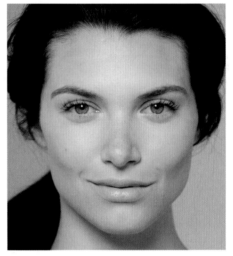

Contouring with bronzer, using Honey

Contour

Apply a contouring color to shape and bring definition to your face. Using a matte color one or two shades darker than your skin, apply contour at the top and sides of your forehead, around the edge of your face, and under your cheekbones and jawline. In the example above, contouring is done with a bronzer color.

Blush

Using a fluffy brush, pat some blush on the center of your cheeks and blend upward toward your ear.

Highlighter

You can apply highlighter either wet, for an intense focus, or dry, with a fluffy brush, to get a subtler sheen. Regardless of whether you apply it wet or dry, you can use highlighter to achieve different effects. Apply it to your cheekbones and around the corners of your eyes to create a crescent shape that frames your eyes. You can create an overall youthful glow by applying highlighter to the center of your forehead, down the bridge of your nose, on your Cupid's bow, and on your chin.

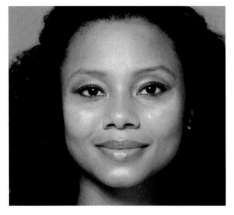

Before blending, crescent shape

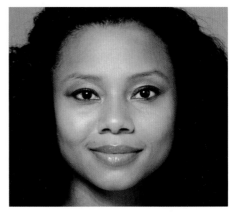

Wet highlighter, using Heatherbelle

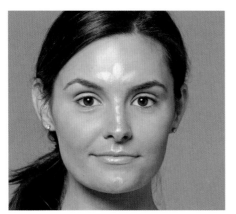

Before blending, dewy look

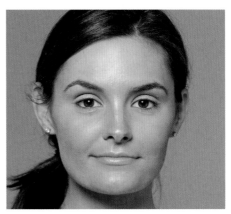

Dry highlighter, using Heatherbelle

Lip Gloss

First apply lip balm to moisturize your lips, then follow up with a lip gloss color. To achieve a pouty lip look, apply either highlighter or a lighter shimmery lip gloss to the center of your lips on top of the first gloss. If you don't have any colored lip gloss on hand, you can mix a little blush into some clear lip gloss, as long as all the blush ingredients are approved for use on lips.

Cupid's Bow
Noun (1567): Two convex curves, usually with recurved ends; the top edge of a person's upper lip

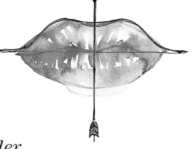

Finishing Powder

Using a large fluffy brush, gently pat the finishing powder over the T-zone, which includes the center of your forehead, bridge and sides of your nose, and your chin. You can also apply the powder anywhere you have used concealer.

CHOOSING COLORS

Once you know the basic application techniques, you will want to choose colors that enhance your natural beauty by complementing your skin undertone, hair color, and eye color. Remember what you learned about color theory in chapter 2.

Skin Undertones

To enhance your skin shade and blend your makeup properly, you must select a foundation that matches your undertone. An easy way to test this is to pick three foundation shades that look close to your skin shade, and apply all three to your jawline. Usually one is too dark and one is too light, while one practically disappears on your skin. Choose that perfectly matched one. You also should choose blushes, bronzers, highlighters, lip glosses, and eye shadows with the same undertone as your skin.

Eyes

When choosing colors for eye makeup, pick tones that work well with your natural eye color. Two popular approaches include using complementary colors to make the eye color "pop," which results in fixing the eyes as the focal point of the face, or using neutral or analogous colors to create a more natural, balanced look. For a refresher on complementary and analogous colors, see chapter 2.

BLUE EYES look best with warm, coppery colors. Try eye shadows in tones of golden brown, warm taupe, copper, warm brown, and golden khaki. Pick eyeliners that are warm brown, taupe, navy, bronze, burgundy, or black.

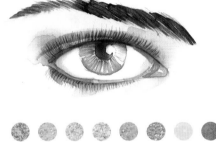

SHADOW COLORS

EYELINER COLORS

GREEN EYES look best with burgundy and violets. Try eye shadows in taupe, eggplant, plum, deep burgundy, lilac, and coppery bronze tones. Pick eyeliners that are burgundy, red brown, eggplant, lilac, violet, warm taupe, or coppery bronze.

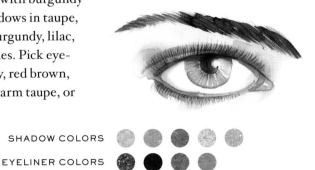

SHADOW COLORS

EYELINER COLORS

BROWN EYES look best with coppery bronze, golden brown, mahogany, eggplant, espresso, indigo blue, dark green, and pewter tones. Pick eyeliners that are black, navy, burgundy, mahogany, eggplant, taupe, bronze, or chocolate brown.

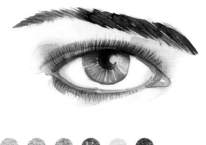

SHADOW COLORS

EYELINER COLORS

GRAY EYES look best with cool shades such as cool brown, burgundy, and silver. Pick eyeliners that are gray, silver, black, purple, or deep brown.

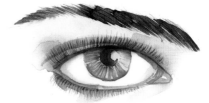

SHADOW COLORS

EYELINER COLORS

HAZEL EYES are a mix of two or more colors. Let whichever one you want to emphasize guide your complementary color decision. For example, if you have green-brown hazel eyes and want to focus on the green, choose colors that complement green eyes. You can also choose universally flattering eye shadow colors or switch it up, wearing colors that flatter the green some days and the brown on other days.

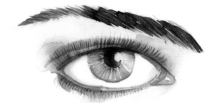

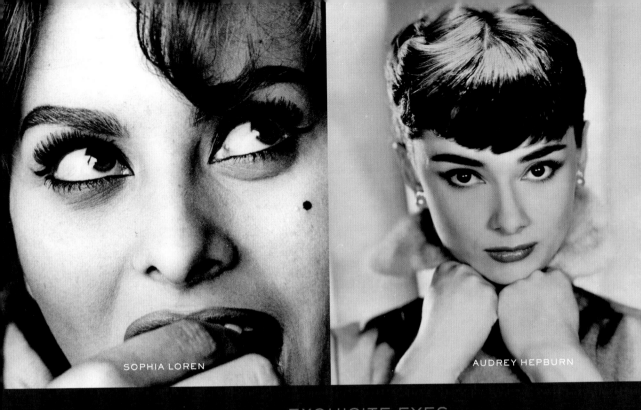

SOPHIA LOREN

AUDREY HEPBURN

EXQUISITE EYES

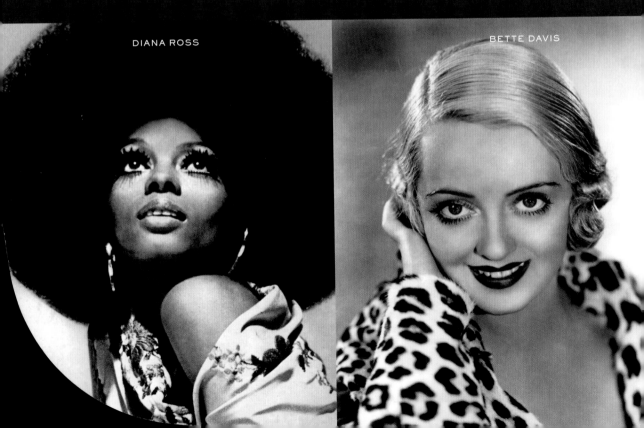

DIANA ROSS

BETTE DAVIS

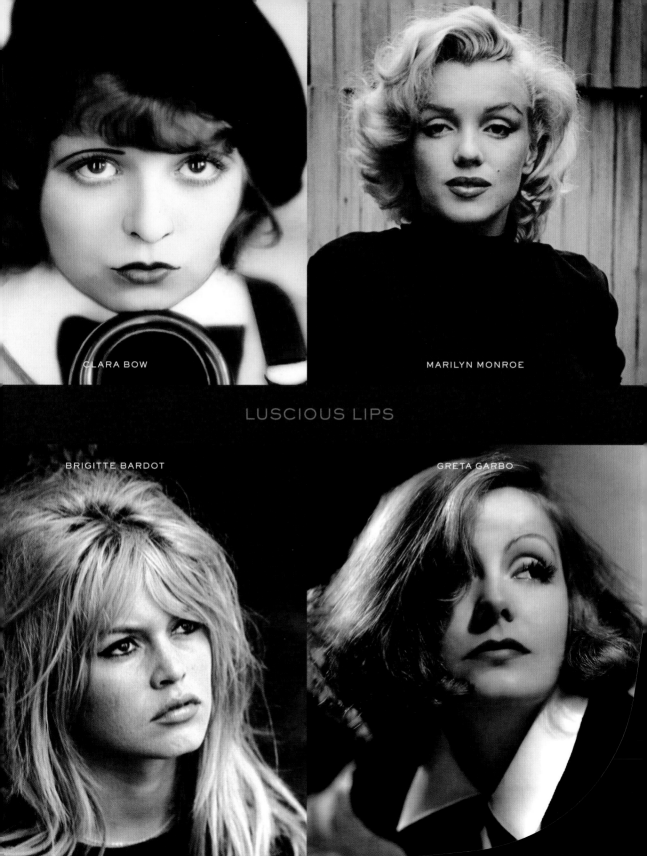

CLARA BOW

MARILYN MONROE

LUSCIOUS LIPS

BRIGITTE BARDOT

GRETA GARBO

LET'S PUT IT ON

Keep two things in mind when choosing colors for your eyebrows: hair color and skin undertones. In general, if you have light hair, choose an eyebrow powder one or two shades darker than your natural hair color. If your hair is dark, choose an eyebrow powder one or two shades lighter than your natural color. If you have warm skin undertones, choose a warm eyebrow powder; if you have cool skin undertones, choose a cool eyebrow powder.

PRO TIP

CHOOSING EYEBROW POWDERS

NATURAL HAIR COLOR		BEST EYEBROW POWDER SHADE
Blonde	◯	One or two shades darker than hair color
Light to medium brown	●	Same color as hair or one shade darker
Dark brown	●	Same color as hair or one shade lighter
Red	●	Same color as hair or one shade lighter
Black	●	One or two shades lighter than hair color
White or gray	◯	Silvery taupe or dark gray

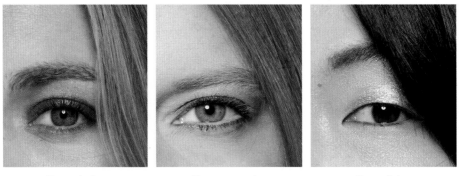

Brows darker than natural hair

Brows same color as natural hair

Brows lighter than natural hair

Face

Bʟᴜsʜ will look most natural when you use the color closest to your cheeks' naturally flushed color. You can easily find this color by lightly pinching your cheeks. For best results, stay in that color family, while also being mindful to match your skin's undertones.

Bʀᴏɴᴢᴇʀ should be subtle. Choose a bronzer two or three shades darker than your natural skin color and with your same undertone.

Cᴏɴᴄᴇᴀʟᴇʀ used to counteract dark under-eye circles should contain hints of yellow. Choosing a concealer one shade lighter than the rest of your face will help brighten the darkness under your eyes. Concealer used to cover blemishes or scars should be the same shade as your foundation.

Cᴏʟᴏʀ ᴄᴏʀʀᴇᴄᴛᴏʀs can be used to counterbalance extreme skin conditions. They work by pairing the color of your skin problem with its complementary color. For intensely red skin, use a green color corrector; for dark circles under your eyes, use a yellow color corrector; for sallow skin, use a light pink or lilac color corrector. Only use color corrector underneath your foundation and concealer.

Hɪɢʜʟɪɢʜᴛᴇʀ should be about three to five shades lighter than your skin color and match your undertones. Cool skin undertones look best with whites, blue or green iridescence, and silvery highlights, while warm skin undertones look best with creams, golds, bronzes, and red or copper iridescence.

Lɪᴘs can be enhanced beautifully with a color two or three shades darker than your natural lip tone.

The goal of using makeup is to enhance the way you look, not to change the way you look.

FIXING THE "FLAWS"

The goal of using makeup is to enhance the way you look, not to change the way you look. But sometimes specific parts of our face make us feel self-conscious, and in those cases it is nice to know a few techniques to help minimize perceived "imperfections."

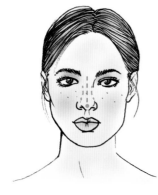

- Apply a light highlight down the bridge of the nose.
- Add a contour color at the bottom of the nose and down each side

wide nose

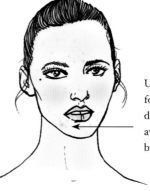

Use a matte foundation to draw attention away from the bumps.

acne

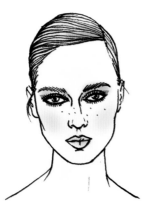

- Dot a light eye shadow in the center or the outer corners of the eyelids.

close-set eyes

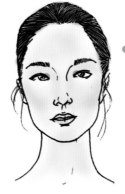

- Dot a light eye shadow in the inner corner of the eyelids.

wide-set eyes

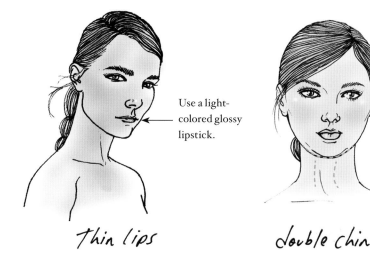

Use a light-colored glossy lipstick.

Brush a contour color under the jawline and down the neck.

Thin lips

double chin

A BALANCING ACT

When creating a look, focus on just one part of the face. Wearing both bright lipstick and dark eye makeup can be too much, so balance things out by choosing one area to spotlight. If you choose your eyes, use dark, pigmented, bright, or sparkly colors to draw attention there, but keep your lips nude or natural. If you instead want to draw attention to your lips, use either rich, dark, or bright colors or glossy and lustrous shades on your lips, while keeping things simple around your eyes with a natural-toned eyeliner, only a little mascara, and no eye shadow. You can also create a balanced daytime look by using medium-toned or neutral colors everywhere, avoiding products that are bold, bright, or very light.

In *Get Positively Beautiful*, one of my favorite books, author Carmindy teaches readers how to accentuate their unique beauty instead of focusing on their perceived flaws. Figure out what you like best about yourself and find ways to draw attention to that feature. Following are some ideas.

SKIN. If you have immaculate, youthful skin, showcase it by skipping foundation entirely or using a foundation with a hint of luster. You could also use highlighter to accentuate different areas of your face, including your forehead, the bridge of your nose, the corners of your eyes, your Cupid's bow, your cheekbones, and under your eyebrows. That glisten will draw attention to your smooth and clear skin, creating a dewy look.

EYES. If you love your eye color, pick colors that complement your natural shade. If you find the shape of your eyes especially attractive, use a dark or bright eyeliner to emphasis that.

EYEBROWS. Make beautiful eyebrows the focal point by shaping them into strong, structured brows and using eyebrow powder.

LIPS. Bright, shiny, and light colors draw attention to lips. If you love your lips, use some bright lipstick or a lustrous lip gloss.

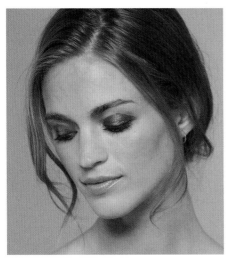

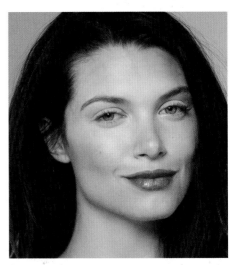

*Spotlight on the eyes
with nude lips*

*Rich color on the lips
with natural eyes*

SKIN CARE AND DIET

Take care of your skin by properly washing, exfoliating, moisturizing, treating, and protecting it with sunscreen. Eat healthfully and stay hydrated to ensure your skin will look its best! I used to apply a lot of products on my skin, but over the years I have found that the fewer products I use, the better my skin looks and feels.

Twice a day I wash my face with a mixture of just water and organic honey — sometimes mixing in a little baking soda as an exfoliator — and then tone with cotton balls soaked in alcohol-free witch hazel. In addition, I use aloe vera for a facial moisturizer. My skin looks best when I get at least eight hours of sleep a night, exercise for at least 20 minutes four times a week, and eat lots of fruits and vegetables, limiting my sugar intake and avoiding most processed, packaged, fried, and fast foods.

Everyone's body is different, and you'll need to figure out what works best for your skin. But pay attention and take care of your skin; it's your largest organ!

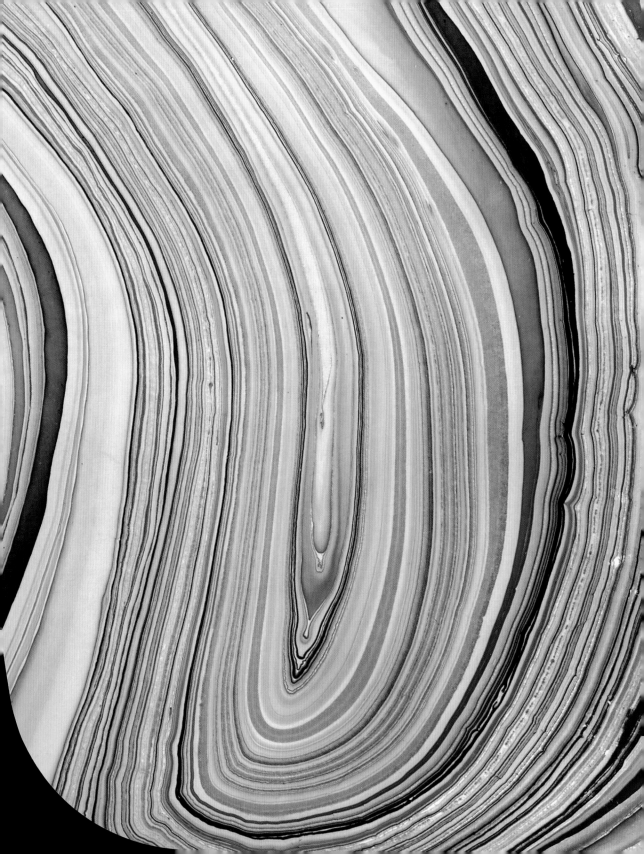

CHAPTER 8

SHARE THE BEAUTY

Perhaps all the dragons in our lives are princesses who are only waiting to see us act, just once, with beauty and courage.

RAINER MARIA RILKE

After creating your own makeup for a while, you may be interested in sharing your cosmetics with others. This chapter gives you a few ideas for how.

HOUSE PARTIES

Before I started selling my products, I invited my family and friends to swatch-and-sample parties. I asked them to test my makeup and give me feedback on my colors and textures. Their honest opinions really helped me improve my products. This kind of gathering was a great low-pressure way to start sharing my makeup with others.

SALES

Eventually you may want to sell your products. In many ways, starting a cosmetics business is no different from starting any small business. For example, you should decide what you want to name your company. Then create a business plan and a budget. There are many books devoted to the topic of starting a business, and plenty of information is available online, too. But because makeup is a personal-care product, with some potential health risks if made unsafely, there are special considerations you will need to keep in mind.

Most important, make sure that your cosmetics comply with FDA rules and regulations. Currently color additives are the only cosmetic ingredients the FDA regulates. For more information on these regulations, see page 230. But be certain you also check www.fda.gov/cosmetics for the most up-to-date rules.

Creating Your Brand

Once you know your products are safe to sell, start defining your brand. Decide who you want your client base to be. Here are some questions to help you through the process:

WHAT COLORS DO YOU WANT TO WORK WITH AND MAKE? Do you want to offer a wide color selection or focus on earth tones, for instance? Do you want to cater your line to women of color? If so, that will influence some of the foundation, concealer, and bronzer colors you create.

WHAT KIND OF INGREDIENTS DO YOU WANT TO WORK WITH? Do you want to specialize in vegan makeup? Are you okay with using some synthetic ingredients?

WHAT TYPES OF PRODUCTS DO YOU WANT TO MAKE? Will you make everything, or will you focus on one product, such as eye shadow?

WHAT PRICE RANGE DO YOU WANT TO OFFER? Do you plan to specialize in making affordable products, or will you focus instead on high-end merchandise?

Next, figure out how you can set your products apart from other brands. Perhaps you want to be known for offering amazing customer service or especially competitive prices or something completely unique, like hand-stamped eye shadows. You might instead decide to identify and then fill a particular hole in the market, such as creating dark makeup that doesn't make women of color look ashy. When it comes to buying makeup, people have a lot of options, so you need to make it clear why someone should consider your cosmetics.

Promoting Your Brand

There are many ways to promote your business and get your name out there, but I recommend starting by making your prices affordable and offering sales. You can increase prices if needed once you build a reputation, but when starting out, you really just want people to try your makeup and cover your costs. Earning a small profit is a bonus.

If someone in the beauty community would be a good spokesperson for your products, don't be afraid to contact her or him. Bloggers, vloggers, beauty gurus, makeup artists, and models regularly work with companies as promoters, reviewers, and brand ambassadors. Start by asking these people if you can send some makeup for them to sample and provide feedback. Never request a positive review. If they love your product, they will want to share it with their followers. But if they don't like your makeup, be respectful of their opinions, ask for any feedback they might have, and work to improve your recipes.

Once your brand starts to grow, reviewers or bloggers may request free samples. You may find that you can't afford to send out a lot of freebies, but you may be able to sell reviewers discounted samples or blogger sample kits, charging only for shipping and the cost of the ingredients. Decide what works best for your company; if you need to, you can decline their request. I have found that if I explain up front why I am not able to offer free samples to potential reviewers, most people respect my honesty and decide to try my products anyway.

TRUNK SHOWS

After hosting a few house parties with friends and family, you might consider having a trunk show. This looks similar to the house parties you may have thrown for friends and family, except that instead of providing samples and collecting input, you will focus on sales and orders. Send out invitations with a couple mini samples a few weeks in advance to get people excited about your show.

Contests and freebies that you advertise in advance are fun ways to encourage people to attend, and you can offer an extra contest entry to anyone who brings a friend. Giving away products doesn't have to be costly for you. Try saving all your experiment batches and extra colors to hand out as free samples.

A makeup demonstration is a great interactive activity at this type of party. Keep it short — under 10 minutes! All you need to cover is what mineral makeup

PRO TIP
YOUR PORTABLE MAKEUP KIT

Whenever you will be applying makeup on others — whether for demonstrations during a house party, craft fair, or convention or as a hired makeup artist — arrive prepared. Come to the job equipped with everything you will need to ensure a perfect look, including your portfolio, face charts, and some pictures of looks you want to achieve. A sizable yet portable makeup case is a must-have. Pack it with a wide selection of foundation shades, concealers, blushes, bronzers, highlighters, eye shadows, and lip colors, along with some makeup remover, facial lotion, and mirrors. Invest in some professional makeup brushes and disposable applicators to make the application as smooth as possible.

Finally, always stress cleanliness! Along with rubbing alcohol to sanitize makeup brushes, bring wipes, hand sanitizer, cotton balls, tissues, and a brush cleaner, which is a mixture of soap, rubbing alcohol, and brush conditioner that you can buy at most makeup or department stores.

is, why it is amazing, and how to use it. Be sure to provide samples for people to play around with. I usually set up a station that offers all my makeup samples and colors, as well as some hand sanitizer, wipes, cotton swabs, and a stand-up mirror.

Having a color chart or containers showing all the colors you offer, a price list, and a stack of order forms handy will help your sales go smoothly. But make sure everyone feels welcome; don't pressure anyone into buying things. You can offer some of your free samples to those who don't want to make a purchase. This will help ensure that everyone leaves with some makeup, which can lead to future sales.

The thing I love most about trunk shows is how intimate and hands-on they can be. Remember, though, that your attendees are potential customers, so keep your business hat on while you're having fun. It's a good idea to get people to pay for what they order that day rather than when you deliver the items. This ensures that you will have enough money to purchase your supplies and guarantees that you get paid. Keep your customers happy: make and deliver their products within a few days of payment. And after the party, send thank-you notes to everyone who came, even if they didn't buy anything!

Craft Fairs and Conventions

When selling at events, make sure you have plenty of products on hand. It is easier to give customers their makeup right away rather than take orders and deliver them later. You can always offer the option of custom orders, but most people will want to buy what you have available.

A short demonstration and/or giveaways will draw customers to your booth. Once you have their interest, ask if they have questions. Let people browse your selection, offering help but giving them space when needed. You won't sell makeup to every person who stops at your table, but hand out as many business cards as possible. Your free samples might prompt people to order from you later.

PRO TIP

CREATING AND RECORDING MAKEUP LOOKS

Keep up with current makeup trends by paying attention to what celebrities wear at events and award shows. Look for celebrities whose undertones, hair and skin coloring, and face shape are similar to yours. Collect pictures of different makeup looks they have worn, and try some out on yourself. I like to keep a pile of makeup books and magazine clippings around my house for inspiration for possible makeup looks. I have even created a binder with pictures I've gathered from books, magazines, and photographs, as well as face charts showing different makeup looks for different occasions.

In addition to collecting your own pictures for inspiration, play around with your makeup to create new looks. You can record these looks by making a simple face chart, applying makeup to the face illustration, and writing down the names and shades you used. If you are a makeup artist, you can store these charts in a binder and bring them with you to makeup consultations, house parties, or shows to serve as a "menu" of looks your clients can choose from.

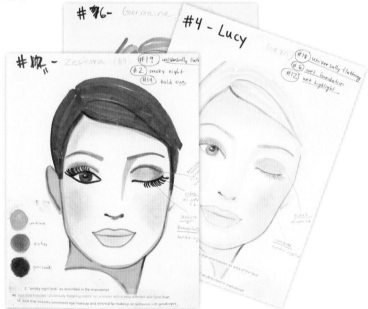

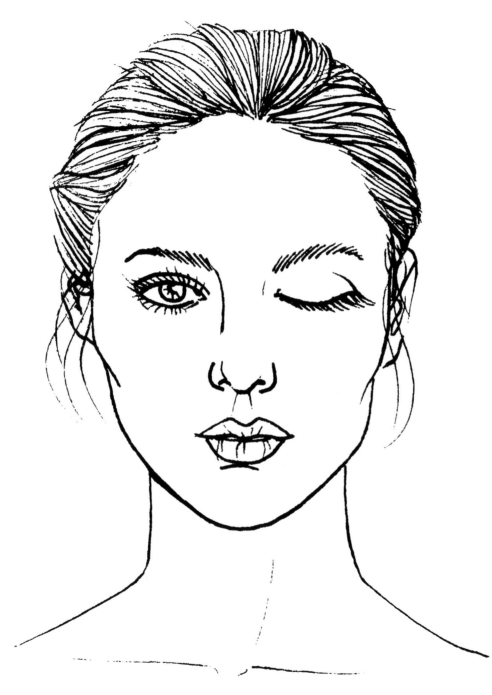

PHOTOCOPY THIS PAGE TO RECORD YOUR OWN MAKEUP LOOKS

Heather is wearing

EYES: Beach Bunny and Stargirl shadows

LIPS: Girl Crush and Basic Lip Gloss mixed with Coral

FACE: Sugar Cookie foundation; Coral blush; Nectar highlighter

Before you sell your cosmetics online, decide whether you want to make your products to order or stockpile them in advance. There are benefits and drawbacks to both approaches. Having a few of each item on hand at all times allows you to ship to your customers faster, but you'll have to spend more money up front, without any guarantee that you will sell all the items you make. In addition, you run the risk of your finished products getting damaged in some way during storage. Alternatively, you can choose to produce only a few samples to show in photographs and then make each product to order. Filling orders will take a little longer if you take this approach but you'll have the benefit of knowing that everything you make is paid for and all the products you ship out are new and pristine.

No matter how you decide to sell your products online, use clear photos accompanied by detailed descriptions that include every ingredient. Take as many photos as possible. Show what the product itself looks like and how the color looks as a swatch on skin. It doesn't hurt to repeat that swatch on a variety of skin colors so customers can get a good idea of how your product will look on them. Finally, remind customers that due to variations in monitors and photography, the color of the makeup they receive may vary slightly from what they see on their screen. Perhaps advise customers to start with a product sample before buying a full-size container.

Carefully pack every item that will ship through the mail, using bubble wrap, tape, and extra padding. Even with careful packing, you should always insure your packages. This will offset the cost to replace an item that gets ruined in transport. Decide on your general and return policies before you sell anything.

Selling through a Vendor

If a vendor is interested in selling your makeup, there are a few different arrangements you might agree to. You can sell to the vendor *wholesale*, offering a discount (usually 5 to 25 percent off the regular retail price) for purchasing a large quantity of your products. Once the vendor has paid you this discounted price, he or she can sell your items directly to customers at a higher price. You may also choose to let the vendor have a *commission* of your sales. In this scenario, you create displays in the shop with products that have not yet been purchased. Whenever one of your items sells, the vendor gets a small percentage of the sale and you get the balance. Finally, some stores will let you *rent* a booth. In exchange for the monthly fee you pay to the shopkeeper, you get all the money from the sales of your products.

Regardless of which arrangement you are considering, be professional, polite, and grateful when meeting with any potential vendor. Bring some products to demonstrate and some to leave with the store owner as a way of saying thanks. In addition to your makeup itself, come prepared with information about your products and about yourself. And make sure that the makeup you are wearing looks perfect, since your face is the best way to advertise your brand.

Bring a binder of information that details your qualifications — such as certification as an aesthetician, dermatologist, or makeup artist — and any experience you might have selling makeup in stores. This file should also include a brief description of each makeup product you sell; a color chart, ingredients lists, and retail and wholesale price lists; and details on why mineral makeup is a great choice for those with sensitive skin. If you can afford to, consider offering store employees a discount for buying your makeup or a commission for selling it. This will encourage them to wear and promote your products.

Once you have an arrangement with a vendor, check on your displays regularly and restock when needed. It's also important to stay with the seasons, changing out your colors to match the current or upcoming trends.

FDA REQUIREMENTS

Whether or not you decide to sell your makeup in the United States, aim to adhere to FDA regulations for makeup application and production. Color additives are currently the only type of ingredient the FDA regulates. For products that you will sell, there are specific labeling requirements as well as rules about batch certification and restricted uses for certain ingredients. Restrictions change over time, so always check the FDA website before you make or sell a batch of cosmetics. It is worth noting, though, that the FDA has no legal authority to approve cosmetics before they are sold. If you plan to sell products outside the United States, check the cosmetic regulations where you will sell, as they may differ from those of the FDA.

Batch Certification

The FDA requires that each new batch of a color additive be checked to verify that it meets identity and specification requirements. Additives subject to batch certifications are known as "coal-tar colors" because the first versions were by-products of processing coal. Today petroleum-based products form the foundation of these "synthetic-organic" colors. These include dyes. If you are using synthetic-organic colorants in your makeup, be sure to get a batch certification number from your supplier. The recipes in this book do not use any pigments that need to be batch certified.

Color additives derived from mineral, plant, or animal sources — including iron oxides, ultramarines, and carmine — are not subject to batch certification regulations. However, the FDA does specify which of these natural colorants are safe for use in which products. Even if you are not selling your makeup, make sure that the colors and particle sizes you use are approved for your desired purpose.

Labeling

All products for sale in the United States must be labeled in compliance with FDA regulations. Each label needs to include the product name and net quantity; the name and address of your business; all ingredients used in the product, in descending order of predominance; the product's intended use; expiration or best-by date; and warning statement, if applicable. Unless you have paid to get your products officially tested, certain claims are forbidden on your labels, including "FDA approved" or a specific SPF rating. To be sure you include all the necessary information on your labels, check the FDA website regularly for new rules.

APPENDIX
INGREDIENTS AT A GLANCE

INGREDIENT	Adhesive	Binder	Color Additive	Healing	Oil Absorbing	Slip	Sheer	Medium	Opaque
	CATEGORY						COVERAGE		
ALLANTOIN				X				X	
ARROWROOT POWDER						X	X		
BEESWAX		X					X		
BISMUTH OXYCHLORIDE						X		X	
BORON NITRIDE	X					X		X	
CALCIUM CARBONATE					X				X
CASTOR OIL		X					X		
CHROMIUM OXIDE GREENS			X						X
COCOA BUTTER		X					X		
COLLOIDAL OATMEAL POWDER				X			X		
CORNSTARCH						X	X		
FERRIC FERROCYANIDE			X						X
FRACTIONATED COCONUT OIL		X					X		
GLYCERIN		X					X		
IRON OXIDES			X						X
JOJOBA OIL		X					X		
KAOLIN	X				X				X
MAGNESIUM MYRISTATE	X	X				X		X	
MAGNESIUM STEARATE	X	X				X		X	
MANGANESE VIOLET			X						X
MICA		X					X		
RICE POWDER				X	X		X		
SERICITE						X	X		
SILICA					X		X		
TALC					X	X	X		
TAPIOCA STARCH						X	X		
TITANIUM DIOXIDE	X		X						X
ULTRAMARINES			X						X
ZINC OXIDE	X		X	X					X
ZINC STEARATE		X				X	X		

| FINISH | | | SKIN TYPE BEST FOR | | | | | | PROPERTY | |
Matte	Semi-Matte/Low Luster	Lustrous	Any	Dry	Oily	Sensitive/Acne Prone	Normal	Not Recommended	Vegan	Botanical
X			X						available, but not all	available, but not all
X					X		X		X	X
	X			X			X			
		X						X	X	
	X				X				X	
X					X	X			X	
		X	X						X	X
X					X	X		X	X	
	X		X						X	X
X			X						X	X
X			X						X	X
X			X						X	
		X	X						X	X
		X		X					available, but not all	available, but not all
X			X						X	
		X		X			X		X	X
X					X	X			X	
X			X						available, but not all	available, but not all
X			X						available, but not all	available, but not all
X			X						X	
	X	X	X						vegan, unless coated with carmine	
X					X				X	X
	X		X						vegan, with no surface treatments	
X					X				X	
	X							X	X	
X			X						X	X
X			X						X	
X			X						X	
X					X	X	X		X	
X					X	X	X		available, but not all	

MICA AND PIGMENT SUBSTITUTIONS MADE EASY

The mica and pigment names used in my recipes are general and descriptive to help you understand what colors you'll be creating. Below is a list of the names I use, paired with some of the names they are sold as by vendors listed in the resources (page 251). I have made every effort to ensure that the alternative colors listed here match as closely as possible what I used in my recipe formulations, but slight variations in your final product colors may occur. See the chart showing the exact colors I used (pages 30–31).

MICAS

NAME USED IN RECIPE	SOLD AS
BRIGHT RED	Hot Step Mama
BURGUNDY	Bordeaux; Colorona Bordeaux; Semi-fine Scarlet
GLIMMERING BROWN BLUE	Chameleon Glitter
GLIMMERING WHITE	Diamond Cluster; Glitter Pearl; Shimmer Pearl; Sparkle Pearl; White Diamond
METALLIC GOLD	Aztec Gold; Gold Aztec; Mayan Gold
METALLIC OLIVE	Crucible Khaki; Metallic Olivia
METALLIC ORANGE	Passion Orange; Peach Sunset
MUTED GOLD	Antique Gold
MUTED SILVER	Antique Silver; Silver Blue
NUDE SILVER	Virgo
PALE YELLOW GREEN	Xian Vistas; Zion's Views
PEACH GOLD	Apricot; Camel; Coral Reef; Golden Peach; Sunstone
PINK BLUE	Winter Rose; Winterveld
SALMON	Bolera; Bolero
SATIN BEIGE	Fine Rose Beige; Mica Beige; Oriental Beige; Soft Beige
SATIN BLACK	Black; Luster Black
SATIN BRONZE	Bronze Fine; Bronze Satin; Fine Rose Tan

NAME USED IN RECIPE	SOLD AS
SATIN BROWN BLUE	Chameleon; Chameleon Fine
SATIN COPPER	Copper Fine; Fine Copper
SATIN GOLD	Fine Saffron; Gold Fine; Mica Gold; Red Gold; Soft Yellow
SATIN SIENNA	Fine Warm Red; Sienna; Sienna Fine
SATIN WHITE	Arctic White; Fine Cool White; Fine White Satin; Icicle; Mica Pearl White; Satin Pearl; Silver Fine; Super Pearly White; White Fine
SILVER GOLD	Limerick
SMOKY BLUE	Blackstar Blue
SMOKY GOLD	Blackstar Gold
SMOKY GREEN	Blackstar Green
WHITE GOLD	Gold Interference; Hilite Gold; Interfine Gold; Iridescent Gold; Pearly Gold Satin; Splendid Gold

PIGMENTS

NAME USED IN RECIPE	SOLD AS
BLACK IRON OXIDE	Black Iron Oxide; Black Oxide Matte Tone
CHROMIUM OXIDE GREEN	Chromium Green Oxide; Chromium Oxide Green
HYDRATED CHROMIUM OXIDE GREEN	Hydrated Chromium Green Oxide; Hydrated Chromium Oxide
MANGANESE VIOLET	Manganese Violet
RED IRON OXIDE	Red Iron Oxide; Red Oxide — Red Shade Matte Tone
TITANIUM DIOXIDE	Titanium Dioxide
ULTRAMARINE BLUE	Ultramarine Blue
ULTRAMARINE PINK	Ultramarine Pink
ULTRAMARINE VIOLET	Ultramarine Violet
YELLOW IRON OXIDE	Yellow Iron Oxide; Yellow Oxide — Matte Tone

INGREDIENTS GLOSSARY

ALLANTOIN

The diureide of glyoxylic acid, a crystal of a botanical extract from the comfrey plant; also can come from the uric acid of cows.
Properties: Moisturizing and skin soften-ing, allantoin offers some skin protection, helps stimulate skin cell renewal and rate of turnover, aids in healing damaged skin, and soothes chapped skin, sunburns, diaper rash, and minor wounds.
Color: White
Coverage: Medium
Finish: Matte
Particle size: 75 microns
Substitutions: Zinc oxide, zinc stearate
Category: Healing
Concentration of use: 0.5%–2% by weight
Skin type best for: Acne, rosacea, eczema, psoriasis, and sensitive skin, but all skin types can benefit from it
Restrictions: None
Notes: Vegan and botanical versions are available.

ARROWROOT POWDER

Starch from various tropical plants, usually *Maranta arundinacea.*
Alternative names: Arrowroot starch
Properties: Lightweight and translucent, arrowroot powder adds slip and a soft feel to minerals.
Color: White
Coverage: Sheer
Finish: Matte
Particle size: 8–50 microns
Substitutions: Cornstarch, tapioca starch
Category: Slip
Concentration of use: 15%–25%
Skin type best for: Normal or oily
Restrictions: None
Notes: Vegan, botanical. Arrowroot pow-der has a shelf life of three to four years if handled and stored properly. It offers poor adhesion to mineral makeup powders.

BEESWAX

A wax produced by honeybees.
Alternative names: Cera alba, yellow wax
Properties: This emulsifier helps stabilize and harden liquid ingredients.
Color: Pale yellow
Coverage: Sheer
Finish: Semi-matte/low luster
Substitutions: Candelilla wax
Category: Binder
Concentration of use: Varies
Skin type best for: Dry or normal
Restrictions: None
Notes: If you want a vegan wax, use candelilla wax. You can buy either bleached or plain beeswax. Bleaching removes beeswax's natural scent and yellow color. It is a good choice if you want a light, odorless wax. If you don't mind the color or scent, I recom-mend sticking with the plain beeswax, as it is less processed.

BISMUTH OXYCHLORIDE

Bismuth is a by-product of lead and copper metal refining that, when combined with chloride and water, becomes bismuth oxychloride, which is used as a cosmetic colorant to produce a pearlized effect.

Alternative names: Bismuthyl chloride, bismuth chloride oxide, chlorooxo-bismuthine

Properties: This pearly powder is dewy and lustrous, offering great adhesion and improving the texture of finished makeup products by giving them a smooth and silky feel. Because it is hydrophobic, bismuth oxychloride is long lasting and will wear well all day, resisting water and sweat.

Color: White

Coverage: Medium

Finish: High luster

Particle size: 6–15 microns

Substitutions: Sericite, boron nitride, mica

Category: Slip

Concentration of use: Less than 98%

Skin type best for: None; see notes below

Restrictions: None

Notes: Vegan. I recommend **not** using this ingredient, as it is a known skin and eye irritant and can cause allergic reactions. It is especially dangerous for sensitive and acne-prone skin.

BORON NITRIDE

An inert mineral in the form of an inorganic powder, made from boron and nitrogen.

Alternative names: Borazon, boron glow, boron mononitride, elbor

Properties: Soft and silky, boron nitride adds slip and improves application. It also absorbs oil, adds adhesion, and provides coverage.

Color: White

Coverage: Medium

Finish: Semi-matte

Particle size: 5–6 microns

Substitutions: Mica, bismuth oxychloride

Category: Adhesive, slip

Concentration of use: 3%–7% in foundation or 5%–40% in eye shadow and blush

Skin type best for: Oily

Restrictions: None

Notes: Vegan. Because it smooths the appearance of wrinkles, boron nitride is great for mature skin.

CALCIUM CARBONATE

Chalk; a powder found in coral, limestone, and marble.

Alternative names: Calcite, calcium salt, carbonic acid

Properties: As an oil and moisture absorber, calcium carbonate helps color retention and improves the adhesion of makeup.

Color: White

Coverage: Opaque

Finish: Matte

Particle size: 3–19 microns

Substitutions: Kaolin, silica

Category: Oil absorbing

Concentration of use: 2%–5%

Skin type best for: Oily and acne prone

Restrictions: None

Notes: Vegan. Use calcium carbonate in small amounts, as it can be drying if it makes up more than 5% of a recipe.

CASTOR OIL

Oil from the beans of the castor plant.

Alternative names: Ricinus communis seed oil

Properties: This thick, lubricating ingredient is often used in lip gloss and lipstick, in part because it remains liquid even at extremely high and low temperatures. When dry, however, it forms a shiny, solid film.

Color: Pale yellow
Coverage: Sheer
Finish: Lustrous
Substitutions: None
Category: Binder
Concentration of use: 50%–60%
Skin type best for: Any
Restrictions: None
Notes: Vegan, botanical. Because castor oil can be drying if used alone, it is best to mix it with another emollient ingredient. When stored and handled properly, castor oil should have a shelf life of at least one year.

CHROMIUM OXIDE GREENS

Chemical compounds made from chromium and oxygen.

Alternative names: Chrome oxide, chromic oxide
Properties: Matte pigment
Color: Deep leaf green; the hydrated version is a teal green
Coverage: Opaque
Finish: Matte
Particle size: Less than 1 micron
Substitutions: Yellow iron oxide mixed with ultramarine blue
Category: Color additive
Concentration of use: Less than 50%
Skin type best for: Any, except acne-prone
Restrictions: Chromium oxide greens are not approved for use on lips in the United States.
Notes: Vegan. Can irritate acne-prone skin.

COCOA BUTTER

Fat extracted from the roasted seeds of the cocoa plant.

Alternative names: Theobroma cacao seed butter
Properties: This emollient ingredient creates a barrier that helps the skin retain its moisture.
Color: Pale yellow
Coverage: Sheer
Finish: Semi-matte/low luster
Substitutions: Shea butter
Category: Binder
Concentration of use: 20%–30%
Skin type best for: Any
Restrictions: None
Notes: Vegan, botanical. Cocoa butter is one of chocolate's main ingredients and is extracted during the process of making cocoa powder and chocolate. It is an extremely stable fat and helps prevent products from going rancid. If handled and stored properly, cocoa butter has a shelf life of at least two years.

COLLOIDAL OATMEAL POWDER

Finely milled whole-grain oats.

Alternative names: Avena sativa kernel flour, oat powder
Properties: An anti-inflammatory skin protectant, colloidal oatmeal powder is soothing to irritated, itchy, dry, or damaged skin.
Color: Light tan to off-white
Coverage: Sheer
Finish: Matte
Particle size: 44 microns

Substitutions: Allantoin, arrowroot powder, cornstarch, tapioca starch
Category: Healing
Concentration of use: 5%–30%
Skin type best for: Acne, eczema, psoriasis, sensitive skin, but all skin types can benefit
Restrictions: None
Notes: Vegan, botanical. Can be a bit gritty when used in cosmetics. Colloidal oatmeal powder has a shelf life of two years when handled and stored properly.

CORNSTARCH
The starch of the corn plant, ground into a silky lightweight powder
Alternative names: Zea mays starch
Properties: This sheer powder adds slip to cosmetics.
Color: White
Coverage: Sheer
Finish: Matte
Particle size: 10–20 microns
Substitutions: Sericite, arrowroot powder, tapioca starch, Dry-Flo, or any other slip ingredients
Category: Slip
Concentration of use: Up to 100%
Skin type best for: Any
Restrictions: None
Notes: Vegan, botanical. If handled and stored properly, cornstarch should keep indefinitely. Cornstarch can be used as a talc substitute but will need added magnesium stearate or boron nitride to give adhesion. Most cornstarch is made with genetically modified corn, but organic, GMO-free versions are available and should be used when making cosmetics.

FERRIC FERROCYANIDE
A matte blue pigment containing iron bound to cyanide so tightly that the cyanide is not released into the final product.
Alternative names: Iron blue, Prussian blue, Prussian blue oxide
Properties: A deep midnight-blue pigment.
Color: Dark blue
Coverage: Opaque
Finish: Matte
Particle size: 0.7–5 microns
Substitutions: Ultramarine blue mixed with black iron oxide
Category: Color additive
Concentration of use: Less than 50%
Skin type best for: Any
Restrictions: Ferric ferrocyanide is not approved for use on lips in the United States. It can be very messy to work with, leaving inky streaks.
Notes: Vegan.

FRACTIONATED COCONUT OIL
A refined version of oil extracted from coconut kernels.
Properties: Fractionated coconut oil is a very light binder that does not clog pores and is easily absorbed into the skin. The process of fractionating makes this oil fully saturated, which results in a very stable product with an extremely long shelf life.
Color: Clear
Coverage: Sheer
Finish: Lustrous
Substitutions: Jojoba oil
Category: Binder
Concentration of use: Varies
Skin type best for: Any

Restrictions: None

Notes: Vegan, botanical. Unlike regular coconut oil, the fractionated version remains liquid at room temperature. If handled and stored properly, fractionated coconut oil has an indefinite shelf life.

GLYCERIN

This natural component of all animal and vegetable fats can be extracted from natural ingredients or produced synthetically.

Alternative names: Glycerol, glycerine

Properties: In cosmetics, glycerin serves as a hydrating solvent that both draws moisture in from the air and holds in the skin's natural moisture.

Color: Clear

Coverage: Sheer

Finish: Lustrous

Substitutions: None

Category: Binder

Concentration of use: Any

Skin type best for: Dry

Restrictions: None

Notes: Vegan and botanical versions are available. Glycerin is a common ingredient used in soapmaking and dissolves in water. Because glycerin can draw up moisture from lower skin layers when used on its own, it is most effective as a moisturizer in combination with other moisturizing ingredients.

IRON OXIDES

Chemical compounds made from iron and oxygen.

Properties: Matte color additives used in foundations and other products.

Color: Come in black, red, or yellow and can be mixed together to make orange and brown

Coverage: Opaque

Finish: Matte

Particle size: More than 100 microns

Substitutions: FD&C dyes

Category: Color additive

Concentration of use: 1%–75%

Skin type best for: Any

Restrictions: None

Notes: Vegan. The natural versions of iron oxides are known as *ochers*.

JOJOBA OIL

Oil extracted from the seeds of *Simmondsia chinensis*, a desert shrub.

Alternative names: Buxus chinensis oil

Properties: This moisturizing binder is an excellent skin conditioner and lubricant.

Color: Golden

Coverage: Sheer

Finish: Lustrous

Substitutions: Fractionated coconut oil, olive oil

Category: Binder

Concentration of use: Varies

Skin type best for: Dry or normal

Restrictions: None

Notes: Vegan, botanical. In addition to controlling mildew, jojoba oil is an effective makeup remover and can be used as a carrier oil. Traditional desert communities have long used it as a leave-in hair conditioner. When handled and stored properly, jojoba oil can have a shelf life of up to five years.

KAOLIN

A soft, white clay made up primarily of kaolinite, a mineral obtained naturally from clay or synthesized, comprised largely of aluminum silicate.

Alternative names: China clay, cosmetic clay, kaolite, nacrite

Properties: Offering oil absorption, adhesion, and coverage, kaolin refines pores, helps with acne as it absorbs excess oil, and serves as an anticaking agent in powders.

Color: White, but also yellow, green, or red, depending on where it is sourced

Coverage: Opaque

Finish: Matte

Particle size: Up to 2 microns

Substitutions: Calcium carbonate, silica

Category: Oil absorbing

Concentration of use: 2%–5%

Skin type best for: Oily, acne-prone, or sensitive skin that does not tend toward dry

Restrictions: None

Notes: Vegan. Use kaolin in low amounts, as it can be drying if it makes up more than 10% of the product. Because kaolinite contains aluminum, those concerned about the aluminum connection to Alzheimer's should avoid it. Although kaolin is not categorized as a color additive by the FDA, because it is available in a range of hues, the color of your final product may vary depending on what kind of kaolin you use.

MAGNESIUM MYRISTATE

A magnesium salt of myristic acid, a saturated fatty acid found in nutmeg, coconut oil, and butter fat.

Properties: Magnesium myristate improves adhesion and slip and also works as a binder, making it easier to press powders into a compact. It helps makeup last longer because it is water insoluble and rub resistant, and it gives makeup a smoother texture and finish and is often used to coat another ingredient to improve its characteristics.

Color: White

Coverage: Medium

Finish: Matte

Particle size: 5–8 microns

Substitutions: Magnesium stearate, zinc stearate

Category: Adhesive, binder, slip

Concentration of use: 5%–10%

Skin type best for: Any

Restrictions: None

Notes: Vegan and botanical versions are available. Magnesium myristate is a great addition to concealer.

MAGNESIUM STEARATE

The magnesium salt of stearic acid, a saturated fatty acid found in beef, coconut oil, and other animal and vegetable fats.

Alternative names: Magnesium octadecanoate, octadecanoic acid

Properties: As an anticaking agent, magnesium stearate improves the slip and adhesion of makeup, giving powders a softer texture. It helps lubricate, bind, emulsify, and thicken powders.

Color: White

Coverage: Medium

Finish: Matte

Particle size: 5–8 microns

Substitutions: Magnesium myristate, zinc stearate
Category: Adhesive, binder, slip
Concentration of use: 5%–10% by weight
Skin type best for: Any
Restrictions: None
Notes: Vegan and botanical versions are available. The vegetable-derived versions have a two-year shelf life if handled and stored properly.

MANGANESE VIOLET

A vibrant pigment made from ammonium manganese pyrophosphate, an inorganic salt.
Alternative names: Ammonium manganese pyrophosphate, mineral violet
Properties: A matte pigment.
Color: Bright violet
Coverage: Opaque
Finish: Matte
Particle size: Less than 1 micron
Substitutions: FD&C dyes or ultramarine pink
Category: Color additive
Concentration of use: Up to 50%
Skin type best for: Any
Restrictions: None
Notes: Vegan

MICA

A range of silicate minerals that can add lustrous color to makeup.
Properties: Mica adds luster, and sometimes color, to makeup products.
Color: Naturally white, but treated with other metals, carmine, and colorants including iron oxides, ultramarines, and titanium dioxide to create a range of colors.
Coverage: Sheer
Finish: Semi-matte to lustrous, depending on particle size
Particle size: 5–150 microns
Category: Color additive
Concentration of use: Varies widely, depending on product and desired effect
Skin type best for: Any
Restrictions: None
Notes: Vegan, unless mixed with carmine for color. The smaller the particle size, the less sparkly the mica will be. To maintain the highest amount of luster in a recipe, mix all the ingredients *except* the mica mechanically, then stir in the mica by hand.

RICE POWDER

Finely ground rice germs.
Alternative names: Oryza sativa powder
Properties: Rice powder absorbs oil, sets makeup, and reduces shine.
Color: White
Coverage: Sheer
Finish: Matte
Particle size: 8 microns
Substitutions: Cornstarch or colloidal oatmeal powder
Category: Oil absorbing, healing
Concentration of use: 1%–9%
Skin type best for: Oily
Restrictions: None
Notes: Vegan, botanical. If handled and stored properly, rice powder has a shelf life up to two years. It can be used as a substitute for cornstarch, and GMO-free versions are available.

SERICITE

A range of silicate minerals ground more finely than mica and left uncolored.

Surface treatments:

- *L-lysine* is an amino acid derived from coconut and palm oils that gives extra cushion in powders, acting as a buffer to separate sericite from the skin. It also helps bind and press powders, making them softer and smoother, as well as oil and water resistant.

- *Silica* acts as a ball bearing, resulting in a smooth finish that helps the sericite slide smoothly over the skin. Powders made with silica-treated sericite are soft and dewy, with extra cushion that gives the makeup a smooth finish.

Properties: Sericite creates a base for mineral makeup, giving it slip and glide, while not noticeably changing the product's adhesion. It reflects light, increases translucency, and gives finished cosmetics a low luster.

Color: White

Coverage: Sheer

Finish: Semi-matte to low luster

Particle size: 5–15 microns

Substitutions: Boron nitride, bismuth oxychloride

Category: Slip

Concentration of use: 5%–75%

Skin type best for: Any

Restrictions: None

Notes: Vegan, with no surface treatments. Sericite is available with other surface treatments in addition to L-lysine and silica.

SILICA

A naturally occurring chemical compound found in quartz, sand, and many living organisms.

Alternative names: Amorphous silica, silicon dioxide

Properties: While wicking moisture away from the skin, silica absorbs oil and serves as an anticaking agent for powder makeup.

Color: White

Coverage: Sheer

Finish: Matte

Particle size: 5–20 microns

Substitutions: Calcium carbonate, kaolin

Category: Oil absorbing

Concentration of use: 1%–15% by weight

Skin type best for: Oily

Restrictions: None

Notes: Vegan. Because silica smooths the appearance of fine lines, it is great for mature skin.

TALC

The powdered form of a hydrated clay mineral, magnesium silicate, which sometimes contains a small amount of aluminum silicate.

Alternative names: French chalk, hydrous magnesium silicate, magnesium silicate hydroxide

Properties: Because talc is hydrated, it offers slip and lubrication to cosmetics while improving adhesion and giving the skin a smooth and soft feel. Talc also absorbs oil and helps control shine.

Color: White

Coverage: Sheer

Finish: Semi-matte

Particle size: 40–50 microns
Substitutions: Cornstarch, rice powder, sericite if using as a base; calcium carbonate or kaolin if using as an oil absorber
Category: Oil absorbing, slip
Concentration of use: Less than 70%
Skin type best for: None; see notes below
Restrictions: None
Notes: Vegan. I recommend **not** using this ingredient, as there is conflicting research linking talc and cancer.

TAPIOCA STARCH

A powder made from the grains of the cassava plant.
Properties: Lightweight and translucent, tapioca starch gives a soft and velvety feel to powders.
Color: White
Coverage: Sheer
Finish: Matte
Particle size: 5–35 microns
Substitutions: Arrowroot powder, cornstarch, sericite
Category: Slip
Concentration of use: 5%–30%
Skin type best for: Any
Restrictions: None
Notes: Vegan, botanical. If handled and stored properly, tapioca starch has a shelf life up to two years.

TITANIUM DIOXIDE

An opaque whitening agent made from the oxide of titanium, which occurs naturally in the minerals rutile, anatase, sphene, and ilmenite.
Alternative names: Titania, titanium (IV) oxide

Properties: Titanium dioxide provides coverage and adhesion for makeup bases while increasing the makeup's opaqueness and protecting skin from ultraviolet light.
Color: Cool white
Coverage: Opaque
Finish: Matte
Particle size: 0.2–0.4 microns
Substitutions: Zinc oxide
Category: Adhesive, color additive
Concentration of use: Less than 60%
Skin type best for: Any
Restrictions: None
Notes: Vegan. Titanium dioxide mined directly from the earth may contain trace amounts of heavy metals. Therefore, most titanium dioxide used in cosmetics has been purified and/or created in a lab to ensure its safety. In addition, most cosmetic-grade titanium dioxide has been micronized to improve application. Some studies have shown that the resulting particles — which are still larger than nanoparticles — are safe for and do not enter the skin. For those especially concerned about the safety of these small particles, nonmicronized versions of titanium dioxide are available, though the coverage and finish of these products will differ from that of the micronized options.

ULTRAMARINES

Pigments composed of sodium, aluminum, silicate, oxygen, and sulfate.
Properties: Matte pigments
Color: Royal blue, purplish pink, or lavender
Coverage: Opaque
Finish: Matte

Particle size: 0.7–5 microns, depending on color
Substitutions: Ferric ferrocyanide (blue) or manganese violet (pink)
Category: Color additive
Concentration of use: 2%–20%
Skin type best for: Any
Restrictions: Ultramarine is not approved for use on lips in the United States.
Notes: Vegan. Because ultramarines contain aluminum, those concerned about the aluminum connection to Alzheimer's should avoid it.

ZINC OXIDE

An inorganic chemical compound made by combining the mineral zincite with oxygen.
Alternative names: Chinese white, flowers of zinc, zinc white
Properties: Adding great coverage, adhesion, and staying power to makeup, zinc oxide whitens pigments and protects the skin from elements and irritants. It reflects UVB rays and offers sun protection. This soothing, astringent, antiseptic, anti-inflammatory, nonirritating substance is FDA approved as a skin protectant.
Color: Warm white
Coverage: Opaque
Finish: Matte
Particle size: 0.1–44 microns
Substitutions: Titanium dioxide
Category: Adhesive, color additive, healing
Concentration of use: 5%–25%
Skin type best for: Oily or normal skin, including acne-prone, rosacea, sensitive skin
Restrictions: None

Notes: Vegan. Cosmetic-grade zinc oxide is offered in micronized and nonmicronized versions. The smaller particles in the low-micron variations offer more transparent coverage while still providing some protection against the sun. However, there is some concern that the smaller particles can enter your skin. I prefer using zinc oxide with larger particles, as it provides more coverage in the final product. In general, all forms of zinc oxide are warmer and less opaque than titanium dioxide, making it a better choice when making foundation for dark skin.

ZINC STEARATE

A metal salt of stearic acid, a saturated fatty acid found in beef, coconut oil, and other animal and vegetable fats.
Alternative names: Zinc distearate, zinc octadecanoate, zinc soap
Properties: Zinc stearate absorbs oil, serves as a binder for pressed powder, and adds some slip.
Color: White
Coverage: Sheer
Finish: Matte
Particle size: 4–7 microns
Substitutions: Magnesium stearate
Category: Binder, slip
Concentration of use: 2%–15%
Skin type best for: Normal, oily, or acne-prone skin
Restrictions: None
Notes: Vegan versions are available.

BASIC GLOSSARY

absorbency. The amount of oil control a powder has.

adhesion. How well a powder sticks to the skin.

aesthetician. A skin-care professional.

analogous colors. Groups of three colors that are next to each other on the color wheel and look harmonious together.

batch certified. Approved by the U.S. Food and Drug Administration for use as a synthetic-organic color additive in food, drugs, cosmetics, or medical devices.

binder (liquid). A fluid ingredient that helps a pressed makeup product hold together.

binder (powder). A dry ingredient that helps a makeup product hold together and keep its shape.

blot. To gently press a tissue to the skin to remove excess oil.

blush. Pink or red makeup that gives cheeks a flushed look.

botanical. Any plant-based ingredient.

bronzer. A medium brown makeup used to give a sun-kissed appearance.

buff. To swirl a product onto the skin with a makeup brush.

carmine. A red color additive made from the insect cochineal.

color additive. A substance used to color a material; pigment.

color corrector. Light pastel makeup that counteracts skin discolorations.

color wheel. A visual guide of the colors and how they interact with and relate to each other.

compact. A small package that holds one makeup product, usually foundation or blush.

complementary colors. Pairs of colors that are located opposite each other on the color wheel. When placed next to each other, they create the strongest contrast possible for those particular two colors and are aesthetically pleasing.

concealer. A skin-tone makeup that helps hide blemishes and discoloration.

contour. A matte powder that is one or two shades darker than the face and used under the cheekbones to give more depth to features and frame the face.

cosmetic grade. Ingredients that are refined enough to be used in makeup products.

coverage. The amount of concealment a product offers.

crease color. A dark eye shadow — usually black, brown, or blue — that is used above the eyelid.

D&C. Stands for *external drugs and cosmetics* and refers to color additives that are subject to batch certification by the FDA.

dash. In cosmetics making, ⅛ teaspoon.

dewy. Having a moisturized and youthful appearance.

drop. In cosmetics making, ¹⁄₆₄ teaspoon.

emollient. Making soft or supple; moisturizing.

FD&C. Stands for *food, drugs, and cosmetics* and refers to color additives approved by the U.S. Food and Drug Administration for use in those products.

finish. The overall appearance of a product.

Food and Drug Administration (FDA). The U.S. federal agency responsible for protecting and promoting public health through regulations and supervision of a variety of activities and products, including cosmetics.

foundation. Makeup that evens out skin color and covers imperfections.

highlighter. Lustrous makeup that is lighter than your face and is used to draw attention to a feature or area.

highlight shade. The lightest color used in the three-color eye shadow application technique.

inert. Cannot harbor bacteria, resulting in no expiration date. Most mineral makeup ingredients are inert.

light scattering. The deflection of a light ray from a single path. In cosmetics, light-scattering ingredients help give the appearance of smoothing wrinkles and fine lines.

lip balm. A creamy, moisturizing lip product.

lip gloss. A thick, shiny, and sometimes colored lip product.

matte. Lacking or deprived of luster, gloss, or shine.

mica. Opalescent colors that are added to makeup to achieve a sparkly appearance.

mid-tone shade. The second color used in the three-color eye-shadow application technique, usually a medium shade.

mixing medium. A clear liquid that is combined with powdered makeup to create liquid or cream products.

MSDS. Refers to *material data safety sheet*. Specifies proper handling and storage guidelines of an ingredient and what to do in an emergency situation involving that ingredient.

opaque. A finish that offers full coverage and allows nothing to show through.

particle size. The length of a powder's particles, usually measured in microns. A larger micron size results in makeup with more luster and less coverage, while a smaller micron size produces more coverage, with a matte finish.

pinch. In cosmetics making, 1/16 teaspoon.

primer. A product that prepares the skin for the application of makeup.

satin. Refers to a finish that is smooth and soft, with little luster.

secondary colors. Tones created by mixing two primary colors together. For example, yellow and blue (primary colors) make green (secondary color).

sericite. A fine-grained colorless mica that is a primary ingredient in mineral makeup bases.

sheer. A finish that is somewhat thin and transparent, which results in products that give a natural appearance.

skin shade. The lightness or darkness of the skin.

skin type. The quality of the skin. The basic skin types are normal, dry, oily, combination, and sensitive.

skin undertone. The color that shines through from beneath a person's skin. It can be warm, cool, or neutral (a combination of the two).

slip. The amount of glide a cosmetic offers. Slip ingredients also lend a sheer quality to products.

smidgen. In cosmetics making, 1/32 teaspoon.

SPF. Stands for *sun protection factor*. Refers to the amount of protection against the sun a product offers.

surface treatment. The coating of a powder with a secondary ingredient.

tad. In cosmetics making, 1/4 teaspoon.

tamping tool. Any instrument used to press powders.

tertiary colors. The colors created by mixing one primary color with a secondary color next to it on the color wheel.

tint. A variation of a color produced by adding white to it.

usage restrictions. The percentage allowed in a finished cosmetic or the application method approved for certain ingredients.

METRIC CONVERSIONS

The measurements in my recipes correspond with how the ingredients and containers are most readily available for sale. If you need to convert US measurements to metric, use the charts below.

WEIGHT

TO CONVERT	TO	MULTIPLY
ounces	grams	ounces by 28.35

VOLUME

TO CONVERT	TO	MULTIPLY
teaspoons	milliliters	teaspoons by 4.93
fluid ounces	milliliters	fluid ounces by 29.57

ACKNOWLEDGMENTS

First, I must thank my husband for being so supportive throughout the process of writing this book. His patience, assistance, and acceptance have helped me in so many ways. Thank you, Clancy, for believing in my talent and for helping me develop into a better version of myself. I also want to thank my two daughters, who truly believe they are making makeup like Mommy while spilling powders all over my desk; they are truly amazing.

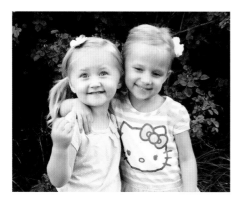

My sincere thanks goes to all my friends and family who have encouraged me to create makeup and write a book, and who have supported me by buying my makeup, investing in my company, and believing in me. I want to thank my sister, Sheila, for always promoting and sampling my makeup; my dad for always advising me in business and being genuinely happy for my success; and my mom for always finding reasons to buy my makeup. Thanks to my friend Julia for friendship, experience, editing skills, and guidance. Also, thank you so much, Heather and Hailey, for letting me sell my makeup in your shop; it was a wonderful experience.

Without the amazing staff at Storey, I wouldn't have been able to write this book. I want to thank Gwen Steege for finding my proposal and believing in my idea. Thank you to my editor, Michal, for helping me present the best book possible, and to Storey's creative director, Alethea, for making it look beautiful. I'd like to thank Mars for taking clear, informative photos, Corey and Jennie for their text production skills, Caroline for turning the unique design into a one-of-a-kind package, and Hartley for making sure the colors on the page accurately reflect my actual makeup products. Thanks also to Sarah, Alee, and Megan for their work marketing and publicizing this book. Many thanks also to the whole crew at the photo shoot in New York: Melinda, Andrew, Tom, and all of the models.

Last, I want to thank those in the beauty industry who have been willing to help me along the way. Thank you, Deb, for introducing me to the world of mineral makeup. Kalia and Kat, from TKB Trading, thanks for your generosity, products, and support.

RESOURCES

INGREDIENTS & PACKAGING

UNITED STATES

DIY Cosmetic Containers
diycosmeticcontainers.com

From Nature with Love
fromnaturewithlove.com

LipBalmTubes.com
lipbalmtubes.com

Making Cosmetics
makingcosmetics.com

Monavé
monave.com

Rustic Escentuals
rusticescentuals.com

TKB Trading
tkbtrading.com
Highly recommended!

CANADA

New Direction Aromatics
newdirectionsaromatics.com

Oshun Supply
oshun.ca

Saffire Blue
saffireblue.ca

Suds N' Scents
sudsandscents.com

UNITED KINGDOM

Aromantic Natural Skin Care
aromantic.co.uk

Gracefruit Limited
gracefruit.com

Specialty Bottle
specialtybottle.com

INGREDIENTS

UNITED STATES

Bramble Berry
brambleberry.com

Ingredients to Die For
ingredientstodiefor.com

Just Pigments
justpigments.com

MicaPowder.com
micapowder.com

UNITED KINGDOM

U-Make It Up
u-makeitup.com

MORE INFORMATION ABOUT MINERAL MAKEUP INGREDIENTS

Cosmetic Ingredient Review
cir-safety.org

Cosmetics Info
cosmeticsinfo.org

Paula's Choice Skin Care Ingredient Dictionary
paulaschoice.com/ cosmetic-ingredient-dictionary

Skin Deep Cosmetics Database
ewg.org/skindeep

U.S. Food and Drug Administration
www.fda.gov/Cosmetics/ ProductsIngredients/Ingredients

INDEX

Page numbers in *italic* indicate photos and illustrations: page numbers in **bold** indicate charts.

TREAT YOUR WHOLE SELF, NATURALLY
WITH MORE BOOKS FROM STOREY

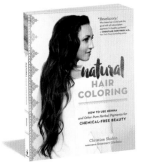

by Christine Shahin

Achieve rich, natural-looking shades of brown, black, red, and even blond by combining henna with three other plant pigments. This accessible guide shows you how to get a variety of stunning hair colors without any chemicals.

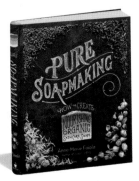

by Stephanie Tourles

Maintain radiantly healthy and beautiful skin, hair, and body with these fun and simple recipes for creams, scrubs, toners, and much more. This wide range of beauty formulas will pamper you from head to toe with nourishing, natural ingredients.

by Anne-Marie Faiola

Make luscious, nourishing soaps with a palette of all-natural ingredients, such as coconut butter, almond oil, coffee grounds, green tea, and much more. Step-by-step photography guides you through every stage of cold-process soapmaking.

JOIN THE CONVERSATION. Share your experience with this book, learn more about Storey Publishing's authors, and read original essays and book excerpts at storey.com. Look for our books wherever quality books are sold or call 800-441-5700.